Metabolism of Anabolic Androgenic Steroids

Author

Victor A. Rogozkin

Professor
Hormone Regulation Department
Research Institute of Physical Culture
Leningrad, U.S.S.R.

CRC Press
Boca Raton Ann Arbor Boston London

Library of Congress Cataloging-in-Publication Data

Rogozkin, V. A.
  [Metabolizm anabolicheskikh androgennykh steroidov. English]
  Metabolism of anabolic androgenic steroids / author, Victor A.
Rogozkin.
      p.   cm.
  Translation of: Metabolizm anabolicheskikh androgennykh steroidov.
  Includes bibliographical references and index.
  ISBN 0-8493-6415-9
  1. Androgens--Metabolism. 2. Anabolic steroids--Metabolism.
I. Title.
  [DNLM: 1. Anabolic Steroids--metabolism.   WK 150 R735m]
QP572.A5R6413   1991
615'.364--dc20
DNLM/DLC   91-15872
for Library of Congress   CIP

International Standard Book Number 0-8493-6415-9

Library of Congress Card Number 91-15872
Printed in the United States

INTRODUCTION

In the general class of steroid hormones, the androgens are among the most important, and for many years they were a subject of thorough study. The detailed investigations of Cochakian, which included a versatile study of the androgenic and anabolic effects of testosterone and its derivatives, led to the creation of a new group of synthetic hormones steroid in nature — anabolic androgenic steroids (AAS).

During several years various AAS were synthesized and were soon widely adopted in clinical medicine.

The discovery, study, and application of AAS are of both great practical and certain theoretical significance. Like other steroid hormones, AAS have become a means of studying metabolic processes in an organism. The discovery of the mechanism of AAS action is inseparably linked with investigations of the molecular-biological principles of steroid hormone action at the level of gene expression. Data on the connection between chemical structure, physical-chemical properties and AAS action, as well as their effect on metabolic processes in an organism, are the basis of a further direct search for new efficacious AAS.

Up-to-date AAS are both an effective remedy and a powerful means of prophylaxis of many diseases. However, like other highly effective hormones, they must be correctly and skillfully used, which requires a knowledge of the mechanisms of their action and possible effects on metabolism in an organism.

The purpose of this book is to collate all AAS investigations that have been accomplished up to the beginning of the 1980s. Such a task is not at all simple since the investigations of AAS and their metabolites are carried out in various fields of science (biochemistry, chemistry, clinical medicine, endocrinology, cattle breeding).

It is quite impossible to examine all the achievements and problems associated with AAS metabolism in detail, without writing several volumes. For this reason we have concentrated on the problems that seem, in the opinion of the author, to be most important, as well as those problems which are within the author's research interests. That is why such problems as the synthesis of AAS, the study of physical-chemical properties of AAS, and some others were not included. The author does not touch upon practical or historical aspects of the problem either since the purpose is to discuss the data which were obtained up to the end of 1985.

The book suggests a method of classifying AAS according to their chemical structure. This classification scheme no doubt suffers from some shortcomings; however it should facilitate the solution of a number of tasks of the book, that is, examination of basic molecular mechanisms of AAS action and selection of physical-chemical methods for the analysis of their content in an organism. The process of steroid intracellular reception plays a major role in the mechanisms of AAS action so long as the selectivity of hormone action is formed just at the stage of their reception by the cell. The book examines some possible mechanisms of a specific AAS interaction with intracellular receptors in various tissues. The formation of hormone-receptor complexes is supposed to be closely connected with energy-dependent processes in the cell. These processes occur through a phosphorylation-dephosphorylation process of the receptor protein. In this regard, the problems discussed directly concern the processes of intracellular metabolism regulation. We have also made an attempt to describe some principal methods of AAS analysis in which the concentration of these hormones in an organism can be controlled.

The author wishes to express his gratitude to the employees of the Hormonal Regulation Department of Leningrad Scientific Research Institute of Physical Culture for their valuable assistance in carrying out mutual investigations, as well as for their help in preparing the manuscript.

THE EDITOR

Victor A. Rogozkin, B.D., is Chief of the Department of Biochemistry and Director of the Research Institute of Physical Culture at Leningrad.

Dr. Rogozkin obtained his training at the State University of Leningrad, receiving the A.B. degree in 1958 and the B.D. degree in biochemistry in 1960. In 1966 he received the D.Sc. degree from the Institute of Physiology from I. P. Pavlov at Leningrad. He served as a Research Associate Professor at the Research Institute of Physical Culture, Leningrad from 1960 to 1966 and as Research Professor and Chairman of the Department of Nutrition at the same Institute from 1966 to 1970. It was in 1970 that he assumed his present position.

Dr. Rogozkin is a member of the All-Union Biochemical Society and the American College of Sports Medicine. He served as a member of the Medical Commission of the International Olympic Committee from 1975 to 1981. He served as Chairman of the Doping Control Committee at the XXII Olympic Games (Moscow, 1980).

Dr. Rogozkin is the author of more than 230 papers and has authored or co-authored six books.

His current major research interests relate to exercise biochemistry and sports endocrinology, especially the metabolic effects of steroid hormones.

TABLE OF CONTENTS

Chapter 1

ANABOLIC ANDROGENIC STEROIDS: STRUCTURE, NOMENCLATURE AND CLASSIFICATION, BIOLOGICAL PROPERTIES

Anabolic androgenic steroids (AAS) are androgen and estrogen derivatives (C_{19} and C_{18} steroids) of a subclass of natural steroid hormones. The AAS structural base is a steran nucleus, a polycyclic C_{17} steran skeleton consisting of three condensed cyclohexane rings in nonlinear or phenanthrene junction (A, B and C), and a cyclopentane ring (D).[1,2] Figure 1 represents a steran ring and a convenient way of numbering carbon atoms.

The basic nucleus has a hard three-dimensional structure. The conformation or "chair" was revealed for cyclohexane rings A, B and C and that of "envelope" or "semichair" for cyclopentane ring D. Free valences of ring-shaped carbonic atoms may be either axial, when they are at right angles to the ring plane, or equatorial when they are on the ring plane (Figure 2).

C_{19} and C_{18} steroids androstane and estrane are parental forms of androgens and estrogen — natural sexual hormones, as well as most AAS (Figure 3).

The structures of androstane and estrane have asymmetric carbon atoms and

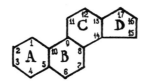

FIGURE 1. Steran nucleus (cyclopentaneperhydrophenanthrene).

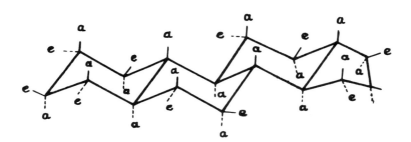

FIGURE 2. Three-dimensional structure of steran nucleus: a, axial group; e, equatorial group.

1

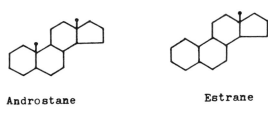

Androstane   **Estrane**

FIGURE 3.   Structure of parental androgen, estrogen and
AAS forms: androstane and estrane.

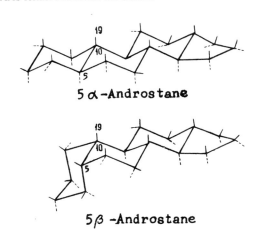

5 α -Androstane

5 β -Androstane

FIGURE 4.   *Cis-trans* isomerism about the A:B ring
junction.

this leads to the existence of isomerides. The isomerides differ in the spatial
location of substituents and in ring junction.[3,4]

As it was agreed, the methyl groups C_{10} and C_{13} have β-configuration and, in
projector formulas, they are located above the molecule plane. Any other
substituents are denoted as "β" if they are situated on the same side and projected
above the plane. The substituents located on the opposite side (below the
molecule plane) are denoted as "α". An intermediate orientation or when the
orientation is unknown is denoted as "ξ". In structural formulas, β, α and ξ are
denoted as a continuous line, a broken line, or a wavy line, respectively.

Cis-trans Isomerism

A hydrogen atom of C_5 may be located either on the same side as the methyl
group of C_{10} or on the opposite side. It is determined by means of the junction of
A and B rings. In the first case, A and B rings are in *cis*-junction when a 5β-isomer
appears and, in the second case, they are in *trans*-junction when a 5α-isomer is
possible[5] (Figure 4).

The modification of parental structures is carried out in several ways:

1. The introduction of carbonyl groups;
2. The introduction of hydroxyl groups;
3. The introduction of double bonds between some two-carbon atoms in a ring;
4. The combination of various substituents;
5. The change of ring structure by means of reducing or increasing the number of carbon atoms.[6]

AAS Nomenclature

Both systematic (rational) and trivial (working) names are widely used.

Systematic names must conform to the IUPAC-IUB 1967 Revised Tentative Rules for steroid nomenclature.[7-9] The last interpretation is given later.[10] The denomination of the parental steroid (androst, estr) is the basis of AAS systematic nomenclature. In systematic nomenclature, prefixes and suffixes are used to indicate the presence of substituents (Table 1).

Any number of prefixes are permitted but only one suffix may be used. Where there is more than one substituent, the suffix is chosen according to the diminution of preference from the list: acid, lactone, ester, aldehyde, ketone, alcohol, amine, ether. Where there is more than one prefix, they are written in alphabetical order. In all cases, the carbon atoms with joined substituents are denoted with figures. The position of a double bond is indicated by the numeration of a lesser carbon atom which is involved in the bond. If there is some alternative, then another carbon atom is indicated in brackets.

If a number of similar substituents exist, "di", "tri" and other prefixes are added before the suffix or prefix.

"Nor" is used as a prefix to indicate the elimination of a methylene group. This results either in a shortening of chain size with the removal of the methyl group or a ring contraction. In the first case, the prefix is preceded by the number of the carbon atom eliminated and, in the second case, by the letter of the ring contracted. The numbering system is modified by means of excluding the highest numbered carbon atom in the ring contracted.

TABLE 1
Common Substituents with Respective Prefix and Suffix Forms

Substituent group	Prefix	Suffix
Double bond (–C=C–)	—	-ene
Triple bond (–C≡C)	—	-yne
Hydroxyl (–OH)	hydroxy-	-ol
Carbonyl (C=O)	oxo-	-one
Acetate (–OCOCH₃)	acetoxy-	-yl acetate
Aldehyde (CHO)	—	-al
Carboxylic acid (COOH)	carboxy-	-oic acid

"Homo" is used as a prefix to indicate the ring expansion. The term is preceded by the letter of the ring expanded.

In the formula, the letter "a" is added to a new highest numbered carbon atom in the ring.

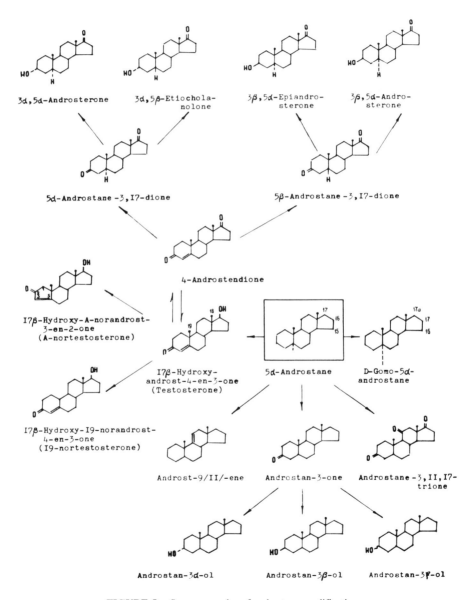

FIGURE 5.   Some examples of androstane modification.

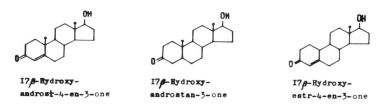

17β-Hydroxy-
androst-4-en-3-one

17β-Hydroxy-
androstan-3-one

17β-Hydroxy-
estr-4-en-3-one

FIGURE 6. Structure of testosterone (left), 5α-dihydrotestosterone (center) and 19-nortestosterone (right).

"Oxa" indicates the presence of oxygen in the ring structure.

Trivial names may be prefixed to emphasize their origin and AAS stereoisomerism. In addition to prefixes used in systematic nomenclature (hydroxy, oxo, etc.) the following are frequently used: "epi" to emphasize the inversion of an asymmetric atom; "dehydro", the removal of two hydrogen atoms from two adjacent carbon atoms or from a carbonyl group; and, "deoxy", the substitution of a carbonyl group by a hydrogen atom. "Dihydro", "tetrahydro", etc. may be used to indicate the addition of a hydrogen to double bonds but not to carbonyl groups. The prefix "allo" (change to 5α configuration) and the symbol Δ^x (unsaturation in position X) may not be used. It should be noted that the same compound often has many trivial names. For instance, 16 names are known for 17β-hydroxy-17α-methylandrosta-1,4-dien-3-one: abirol, C-17309, danabol, dehydroxymethyltestosterone, dianabol, dianavit, deabol, methandienone, methandrostenolone, methylhydroxyandrostadionone, nabolin, NBL, nerobol, neroboletta, stenolon, and vanabol.[11] Such names may not be used in the title or in the summary.

Some forms of the modification of a parental androstane structure are given in Figure 5.

AAS Biological Properties

Among some natural steroids, 17β-hydroxy-androst-4-en-3-one (testosterone) and its derivatives 5-dihydrotestosterone and 19-nortestosterone (male sex hormones synthesized in Leydig cells of testicles and adrenals) are most similar to AAS structurally (Figure 6).

The biological activity of testosterone and some of its derivatives is manifested in androgenic and anabolic action. The androgenic effect is stipulated mainly by the presence of a 17-hydroxyl group. In the absence of 17-oxygen function, as in 4,16-androstandien-3-one, the androgenic activity is completely lost.[12] By the oxidation of the 17β-hydroxyl group with the formation of 17-oxo-steroids (5α-androstane-3α,17β-diol), the androgenic activity is considerably reduced or disappears.[13] The conformation of ring A is of great significance too. The presence of a double bond in position C_4-C_5 stipulates the reduction of C_4-C_5 double bond with the combination of a hydrogen atom in position 5 (as in 5α-dihydrotestosterone). This leads to the formation of the conformation "chair" which considerably intensifies androgen properties of the steroid.[14]

3-Oxo group is also necessary for androgen activity. 5α-Androsta-3β,17β-diol has 60% of the testosterone activity, though in this case the 17β-OH group remains.[13] A reduction of testosterone androgenic properties however is possible. It occurs by introducing an additional double bond into ring A which leads to ring flattening. Coincidentally, the removal of the 10-methyl radical (C_{19}) greatly reduces androgenic properties.[14]

The analysis of the structure of natural steroid functional organization created the basis for a directed synthesis of artificial hormones with various biological activities.

During AAS synthesis by means of a testosterone chemical modification, 5α-dihydrotestosterone and 19-nortestosterone seek first to raise the anabolic capability of the molecule and, second, to reduce the velocity of its metabolism by injection into the organism in order to obtain the highest anabolic effect at a low steroid concentration.

One may distinguish four types of modifications in testosterone, and its derivatives 5α-dihydrotestosterone and 19-nortestosterone, as they are most frequently seen during AAS synthesis:

1. Modification of C_{17}:
    a. Esterification by carboxylic acids or by other radicals (17β-OH[R]);
    b. Oxidation of 17β-OH in 17-keto;
    c. Isomerization of 17β-OH in 17α-OH;
    d. Alkylation (17α-CH$_3$; 17α-C$_2$H$_5$).
2. Modification of C_3:
    a. Reduction of 3-keto in 3α-OH or 3β-OH and its esterification;
    b. Elimination of 3-keto group.
3. Modification of ring structure:
    a. Dehydrogenation — an introduction of additional double bonds;
    b. Introducing oxygen into ring A;
    c. Dislocation of double bonds;
    d. Ring A junction with other ring structures.
4. Hydrogen substitution of C_1, C_2, C_4, C_7, C_9, C_{13} and C_{17} by different radicals (C1, F, OH, CH$_3$, CHO and others).

More than 120 AAS have been synthesized and produced since 1980. It has become necessary to create a standardized classification system of these hormones. In 1975 Camerino and Sciaky[15] examined the structure of 28 AAS and divided them into two groups: the derivatives of androstane and those of 19-norandrostane (estrane). In each group the presence of steroids having: (a) OH-group (free and esterified) in 17β-position and a hydrogen atom in 17α-position and (b)17β-OH group and 17α-alkyl group (methyl and ethyl) was noted.

The substances of group "a" are active only by parenteral introduction, while the steroids of "b" are used both orally and parenterally. The type of acid used by the esterification of the 17β-OH group established the duration of AAS action. According to this classification the division of 28 AAS was accomplished.

The other classification offered by Pivnitsky[16] divides AAS into three groups and is based on the chemical structures of testosterone, 5α-dihydrotestosterone and 19-nortestosterone.

In 1979, on the grounds of the analysis of 91 AAS structures, we offered the classification which includes not only the division into 3 series according to the structure of parental forms (androstane, androstene and estrane), but also according to the character of the modified parental forms of C_{17}, C_3 and ring structures.[17] The modifications include the hydrogen substitution of C_1, C_2, C_4, C_7, C_9, C_{13} and C_{17} by different radicals basically establishing the isolation of contracts (Tables 2 to 4).

The division of numerous AAS specimens into series, contracts and subcontracts proved to be essential while developing fast quantitative methods of determining their content in various biological fluids in organic tissues. It has enabled investigators to plan some systematic methods of studying the metabolism of this large group of steroid hormones.

The biological activity of AAS is evaluated according to their anabolic and androgenic activities.

The androgenic activity of steroids is determined by increased weight of the ventral prostate (v.p.) or seminal vesicles (s.p.). Since v.p. and s.p. react on various AAS unequally, that is v.p. reacts stronger on one preparation than s.p., we have expressed the androgenic activity as the average reaction of both organs.[16,18]

The anabolic activity of synthetic AAS is evaluated in several ways: nitrogen balance (protein anabolic activity)[19] and the growth weight of the kidney (renotrophic activity) are two examples.[20] The method of determining myotrophic activity by growth weight, in m. levator ani (m.l.a.) of rats, has been practiced on a large scale.[21,22] However, the m.l.a. increase test has some limitations, as long as the growth stimulation is caused by not only anabolic activity, but also by androgenic effects of the steroids.[23-25]

A qualitative estimation of synthesized AAS anabolic and androgenic effects, based on well-known methods, does not meet any difficulties. The complications occur with the qualifying of a new AAS anabolic and androgenic activity, which is rather important for revealing the expediency of diverse chemical modifications in a new steroid molecule.

The expression of AAS activity as the ratio of studied and standard steroid doses, which are necessary for obtaining the same reactions of the organ tested, does not give accurate relative values. This is due to a lack of parallelism of the dose curves during the estimation of AAS action. To obtain the data on relative activities, for fixed doses or doses causing organ weight doubling in comparison with the control, minimum doses causing growth in m.l.a. weight by 50% are usually used.[26-29]

TABLE 2
Anabolic Androgenic Steroids of Androstane Series 5α

Subseries	Sub-subseries	Basic chemical structure of subseries	Basic chemical radicals	Names — Systematic	Names — Trivial
I	1		3-oxo;17β-OH(R)	17β-hydroxyandrostan-3-one	Androstanolone (dihydro-testosterone)
				17β-[(1-oxopentyl)oxy]-androstan-3-one	-valerionate
				17β-(1-oxopropoxy)-androstan-3-one	-propionate
				17β-[(oxopentyl)oxy]-androstan-3-one	-enantate
				17β-(benzoyloxy)-androstan-3-one	-benzoate
	2		+2α-R	17β-hydroxy-2α-methyl-androstan-3-one	Drostanolone
				17β-(1-oxopropoxy)-androstan-3-one	-propionate
	3		+17α-CH₃	17β-hydroxy-17α-methyl-androstan-3-one	Mestanolone
	4		+1α-CH₃	17β-hydroxy-1α-methyl-androstan-3-one	Mesterolone
	5		+1α-CH₃; 17α-CH₃	17β-hydroxy-1α,17α-dimethyl-androstan-3-one	Dimethylandrostanolone
II	1		1-en; 3-oxo; 17β-OH(R)	17β-[(1-methoxycyclohexyl)-oxy]-androst-1-en-3-one	Mezabolone

	2		+1-CH₃	17β-hydroxy-1-methylandrost-1-en-3-one	Metenolone -anantate
	3		+2-CH₃	17β-[(1-oxoheptyl)oxy]-1-methylandrost-1-en-3-one 17β-[(acetyl)oxy]-1-methyl-androst-1-en-3-one	-acetate
III	1		3β-OH;17β-OH; 17α-CH₃	17α-methylandrostane-3β,17β-diol	Methylandrostanediol
IV	1		3α-OH; 17β-OH	Androstane-3α,17β-diol	Androstanediol
V	1		3α-OH; 17-oxo	3α-hydroxyandrostan-17-one	Androsterone

TABLE 2 (continued)
Anabolic Androgenic Steroids of Androstane Series 5α

Subseries	Sub-subseries	Basic chemical structure of subseries	Basic chemical radicals	Names Systematic	Names Trivial
VI	1		2-oxa; 3-oxo; 17β-OH; 17α-CH₃	17β-hydroxy-17α-methyl-2-oxa-androstan-3-one	Oxandrolone
VII	1		17β-OH; 17α-CH₃; (3,2-C)-pyrazol; isoxazol; (2,3-C)-(1,2,5)-oxadiazol and other cyclic structures	17α-methylandrostano-(2,3-C)-(1,2,5)-oxadiazol-17β-ol / 17α-methylandrostan-(3,2-C)-isoxazol-17β-ol / 17α-methyl-2'H-androst-2-eno-(3,2-C)-pyrazol-17β-ol	Furazabol / Androisoxazol / Stanozolol
VIII	1		3-oxo 2; 17β-OH; 17α-CH₃	17β-hydroxy-2-hydroxy-methylene-17α-methyl-androstan-3-one	Oxymetholone

IX

1

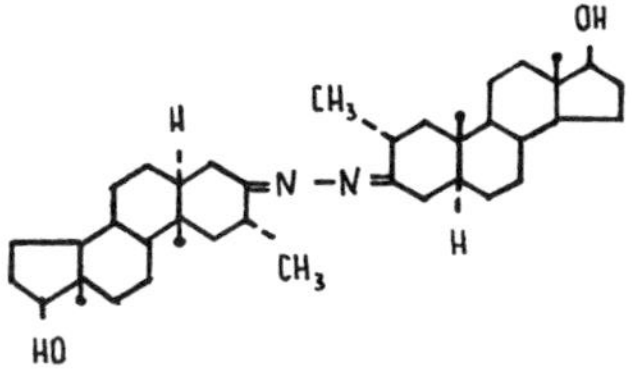

17β-OH(R); 2α-CH₃; 3-yliden-hydrazone

17β-OH(R); 2α-CH$_3$; 3-yliden-hydrazone

17β-hydroxy-2α-methyl-androstan-3-yliden (17β-hydroxy-2α-methyl-androstan-3-yliden)-hydrazone — Bolazine

2α-methyl-17β-[(1-oxo-hexyl)oxyandrostan-3-yliden-2α-methyl-17β-[(1-oxohexyl)oxy]-androstan-3-yliden]-hydrazone — Caproate

+17α-CH₃

+17α-CH$_3$

17β-hydroxy-2α, 17α-dimethylandrostan-3-yliden-(17β-hydroxy-2α,17α-dimethylandrostan-3-yliden)-hydrazone hydrazone — Mebolazine

TABLE 3
Anabolic Androgenic Steroids of Androstene Series

Subseries	Sub-subseries	Basic chemical structure of subseries	Basic chemical radicals	Names Systematic	Trivial
I	1	OH(R)	3-oxo; 4-ene; 17β-OH(R)	17β-hydroxyandrost-4-en-3-one	Testosterone
				17β-(acetyloxy)-androst-4-en-3-one	-acetate
				17β-[(cyclohexylcarbonyl)-oxy]-androst-4-en-3-one	-cyclohexyl-carboxylate
				17β-(cyclohexylacetoxy)-androst-4-en-3-one	-cyclohexyl-acetate
				17β-(3-cyclohexyl-1-oxo-propoxy)-androst-4-en-3-one	-cyclohexyl-propionate
				17β-(3-cyclopentyl-1-oxo-propoxy)-androst-4-en-3-one	-cyclopentyl-propionate
				17β-[(1-oxyheptyl)oxy]-androst-4-en-3-one	-enantate
				17β-[(cyclohexylcarbonyl)oxy]-androst-4-en-3-one	-hexahydro-benzoate
				17β-[3-[4-(hexyloxy)phenyl]-oxopropoxy]-androst-4-en-3-one	-hexyloxy-phenylpropionate
				17β-[(1,3-dioxododecyl)oxy]-androst-4-en-3-one	-oxolaurate
				17β-[(1-oxo-4-methylpentyl)oxy]-androst-4-en-3-one	-methylpentanoate

No.	Substituent	Systematic name	Common name
		17β-[(3-pyridinecarbonyl)oxy]-androst-4-en-3-one	-nicotinate
		17β-[(phenylacetate)oxy]-androst-4-en-3-one	-phenylacetate
		17β-(1-oxo-3-phenylpropoxy)-androst-4-en-3-one	-phenylpropionate
		17β-(1-oxopropoxy)-androst-4-en-3-one	-propionate
		17β-(1-oxoundecyloxy)-androst-4-en-3-one	-undecanoate
		17β-[(trimethylsilyl)-oxy]-androst-4-en-3-on	Silandrone
		17β-[1(hydroxy)-2,2,2-trichlor-ethoxy]-androst-4-en-3-one	Chlorotestosterone
		17β-[(1-acetyloxy)-2,2,2-trichlorethoxy]-androst-4-en-3-one	-acetate
2	+17α-CH$_3$	17β-hydroxy-17α-methyl-androst-4-en-3-one	Methyltestosterone
3	+4-Cl	4-chloro-17β-hydroxyandrost-4-en-3-one	Chostebol
4	+4-OH; 17α-CH$_3$	4,17-dihydroxy-17α-methyl-androst-4-en-3-one	Oxymesterone
5	+4-Cl; 11-OH(R); 17α-CH$_3$	4-chlor-11β,17β-dihydroxy-17α-methylandrost-4-en-3-one	Chloroxymesterone
	+9α-F; 11β-OH; 17α-CH$_3$	9α-fluoro-11β,17β-dihydroxy-17α-methylandrost-4-en-3-one	Fluoxymesterone (Galotestin)
7	+7α-CH$_3$; 17α-CH$_3$	17β-hydroxy-7α,17α-dimethyl-androst-4-en-3-one	Bolasterone (7,17-dimethyl-testosterone)

TABLE 3 (continued)
Anabolic Androgenic Steroids of Androstene Series

Subseries	Sub-subseries	Basic chemical structure of subseries	Basic chemical radicals	Systematic	Trivial
					Names
II	8		$+1\alpha,7\alpha$-diacetylthio; 17α-CH$_3$	$1\alpha,7\alpha$-bis(acetylthio)-17β-hydroxy-17α-methylandrost-4-en-3-one	Thiomesterone
	1		3-oxo; 1,4-diene; 17β-OH(R)	17β-(cyclopenten-1-yloxy)-androsta-1,4-dien-3-one	Quinbolone
				17β-hydroxyandrosta-1,4-dien-3-one	Boldenone
	2		$+17\alpha$-CH$_3$	17β-hydroxy-17α-methyl-androsta-1,4-dien-3-one	Methandienone (methandro-stenolone, dianabol and others)
	3		+4-OH or 4-Cl; 17α-CH$_3$	$4,17\beta$-dihydroxy-17α-methyl-androsta-1,4-dien-3-one	Enestebol
				4-chloro-17β-hydroxy-17α-methylandrosta-1,4-dien-3-one	Dehydrochlormethyl-testosterone
	4		+4-Cl; 11β-OH(R); 17α-CH$_3$	4-chloro-11β,17β-dihydroxy-17α-methylandrosta-1,4-dien-3-one	Chloroxydienone
	5		$+2$-C$\overset{\text{O}}{\underset{\text{H}}{=}}$; 11α-OH; 17α-CH$_3$	$11\alpha,17\beta$-dihydroxy-17α-methyl-3-oxo-androsta-1,4-dien-2-carboxaldehyde	Formebolone

		Structure	Substituents	Systematic name	Common name
III	1		3β-OH(R); 5-ene; 17-oxo	3β-hydroxyandrost-5-en-17-one	Prasterone
IV	1		3β-OH(R); 3,5-diene; 17β-OH; 17α-CH$_3$	3β-(cyclopentyloxy)-17α-methylandrosta-3,5-dien-17β-ol	Penmestrol
				3β-hexyloxy-17α-methyl-androsta-3,5-dien-17β-ol	Hexoxymestrol
	2		3β-OH(R); 17β-OH; 5-ene	androst-5-ene-3β,17β-diol-dipropionate	Androstenediol-dipropionate
			3β-OH(R); 17β-OH(R); 5-ene	17α-methylandrost-5-ene-3β,17β-diol	Methandriol
			3β-OH(R); 17β-OH(R); 5-ene; 17α-CH$_3$	17α-methylandrost-5-ene-17β-acetate-3β,17β-diol-bis-(3-oxononanoate)	-bisenanthoyl-acetate
				17α-methylandrost-5-ene-3β,17β-dioldipropionate	-dipropionate
				17α-methylandrost-5-ene-3β,17β-diol-3-propionate	-propionate
V	1		(3,2-C)-pyrazol:4-ene; 17β-OH(R); 17α-CH$_3$	17α-methylandrost-4-ene-(3,2-C)-pyrazol-17β-ol	Hydroxystenozol

TABLE 4
Anabolic Androgenic Steroids of Estrene Series

Subseries	Sub-subseries	Basic chemical structure of subseries	Basic chemical radicals	Names Systematic	Names Trivial
1	1		3-oxo; 4-ene; 17β-OH(R)	17β-hydroxyestr-4-en-3-one	Nandrolone
				17β-[(1-oxohexyl)-oxy]-estr-4-en-3-one	-capronate
				17β-(3-cyclohexyl-1-oxo-propoxy)-estr-4-en-3-one	-cyclohexylpropionate
				17β-(3-cyclopentyl-1-oxopropoxy)-estr-4-en-3-one	-cyclopentylpropionate
				17β-[[(4-methylbicyclo[2.2.2]-oct-2-en-1-yl)carbonyl]oxy]-estr-4-en-3-one	-cyclotate
				17β-[(1-oxodecyl)-oxy]-estr-4-en-3-one	-decanoate (retabolyl)
				17β-[-3-(2-furanyl)-1-oxo-propoxy]-estr-4-en-3-one	-furylpropionate
				17β-[(cyclohexyl-carbonyl)oxy]-estr-4-en-3-one	-hexahydrobenzoate
				17β-[3]-(hexyloxy)-phenol]1-oxopropoxy]-estr-4-en-3-one	-hexyloxyphenylpropionate
				17β-(3-carboxy-1-oxo-propoxy)-estr-4-en-3-one	-hydrogensuccinate
				17β-[(1-oxododecyl)-oxy]-estr-4-en-3-one	-laurate

No.	Substituents	Structure	Name
		17β-(1-oxo-3-phenylpropoxy)-estr-4-en-3-one	-phenylpropionate (durabolin, nerabolyl, phenobolyl)
		17β-(1-oxopropoxy)-estr-4-en-3-one	-propionate
		17β-[(1-oxoundecyl)-oxy]-estr-4-en-3-one	-undecylate
		17β-[(tricyclo[3.3.1^{7,3}]-dec-1-yl-carbonyl)-oxy]-estr-4-en-3-one	Bolmantalate
2	+17α-CH$_3$	17β-hydroxy-17α-methylestr-4-en-3-one	Methylnortestosterone
3	+4-OH or 4-Cl	17β-(3-cyclopentyl-1-oxo-propoxy)-4-hydroxy-estr-4-en-3-one	Oxaboloncypionate
		4-chloro-17β-hydroxy-estr-4-en-3-one	Norclostebol
		4-chloro-17β-(acetyloxy)-estr-4-en-3-one	-acetate-17
4	17α-CH$_3$; 4-OH or 4-Cl	4-chloro-17β-hydroxy-17α-methyl-estr-4-en-3-one	Chlordrolone
5	+7α-CH$_3$	17β-hydroxy-7α-methylestr-4-en-3-one	Trestolone
		17β-(acetyloxy)-7α-methyl-estr-4-en-3-one	-acetate
6	+7α-CH$_3$; 17α-CH$_3$	17β-hydroxy-7α,17α-dimethyl-estr-4-en-3-one	Mibolerone
7	+17α-C$_2$H$_5$	17β-hydroxy-17α-ethylestr-4-en-3-one	Norethandrolone (nilevar)
		17α-ethylestr-4-en-17β-ol	Ethylestrenol (orabolin, maxibolin)

TABLE 4 (continued)
Anabolic Androgenic Steroids of Estrene Series

Subseries	Sub-subseries	Basic chemical structure of subseries	Basic chemical radicals	Names	
				Systematic	Trivial
II	1		3β-OH; 17β-OH(R); 4-ene	estr-4-ene-3β,17β-diol	Bolandiol
				estr-4-ene-3β,17β-diol-dipropionate	-dipropionate
III	1		3β-OH; 17α-OH; 4-ene	estr-4-ene-3β,17α-diol-3-propionate	Propetandrol
IV	1		17β-OH; 5-ene; 17α-ethyl	17α-ethyl-estr-5-ene-17β-ol	Bolenol

V	1	 3-oxo; 17α-OH; 2-oxa; 5[10]-ene	17α-hydroxy-7α-methyl-estr- -5[10]-en-2-oxa-3-one	Tibolone
VI	1	 3-oxo; 17β-OH; 4,9,11-triene	17β-hydroxy-estra-4,9,11-trien- 3-one	Trenbolone
			17β-acetyloxy-estra-4,9,11- trien-3-one	-acetate
			17β-(hexahydrobenzylcarboxy)- estra-4,9,11-trien-3-one	-hexahydrobenzylcarbonate
	2	+17α-CH₃	17β-hydroxy-17α-methylestra- 4,9,11-trien-3-one	Metribolone
VII	1	 3-oxo; 4-ene; 17β-OH; 13α-C₂H₅; 17α-C₂H₅	17β-hydroxy-13α,17α-diethyl- estr-4-en-3-one	Norboletone

For an integral evaluation of hormone anabolic properties the anabolic index is used. It is characterized by the ratio of myotrophic activity to androgenic activity. An anabolic index greater than one indicates a steroid to be anabolic in nature, while an index less than one represents an androgenic steroid.

While estimating the anabolic effect of various AAS it should be taken into consideration that there exists a maximum anabolic effect or a certain limit in which increasing the steroid dose or changing its chemical structure has no effect. In experiments on rats a tripling of m.l.a. weight growth may be obtained, and by determining the nitrogen balance in men, nitrogen retention may reach 23%. While estimating the anabolic effect (100%), these values may be taken as finite, and on this basis one may express the anabolic potential of AAS investigated as a percentage. Such an approach shows that there exists practical possibilities and hidden reserves in increasing the AAS anabolic effectiveness.

While analyzing the bonds of anabolic and androgenic activities, a large series of comparative investigations carried out under identical conditions may be the most reliable ones. However in this case the results may only be considered to be half-quantitative.[16] Such comparative investigations of a large number of synthesized AAS have not been carried out. The findings of 20 works on the estimation of androgenic and anabolic activity in 19 AAS were analyzed in a review.[30]

Recently some attempts have been made to create a new way for expressing the anabolic activity and the anabolic index of steroids. A graphic description of the myotrophic/androgenic ratio is a good example. It is accomplished on the basis of a determination of the content of the nucleic acids and the ratios of RNA/DNA in seminal vesicles and m.l.a. in grown-up castrated rats after injecting different doses of 19-nortestosterone.[31] The offered method takes into account not only the metabolic state in these two organs, but also the AAS content in blood. A close correlation between steroid receptor binding sites and the 19-nortestosterone biological effect was demonstrated.

17α-Steroids alkylation — methyl and ethyl — substitution in 17α-position makes a valuable contribution to the increase of AAS anabolic effects. The efficiency of the action of 17α-alkylated steroids is associated with the increase of their stability to oxidation and the conversion to low active 17-keto steroids. The alkylation according to position 17 results from the fact that in the process of intracellular metabolism the transformation of this part of the steroid does not take place. In this case it is necessary to underline the possible disturbance in liver metabolism which is due to the presence of alkyl groups in AAS 17α-position.

The esterification of the 17β-hydroxyl group by carboxylic acids increases the steroid activity due to the prolongation of its action. By esterification, the steroid gets lipophilic properties and the capability of retaining fat tissue. By the migration from fat depot to blood, its hydrolysis by plasma enzymes, with the release of an active form with free 17β-OH group, occurs. The release velocity from the depot depends on the length of the carboxylic acid carbon chain. This modification has no effect on the anabolic index. It only leads to a relative increase of the activity by injection into the organism. It was shown that the anabolic activity of 19-nortestosterone derivatives, esterified by 17-hydroxyl group 17β-(1-oxodecyloxy)-estr-4-en-3-one, 17β-(1-oxo-3-phenylpropoxy)-estr-4-en-3-one), gradually developed and was maintained at a high level for a long period of time.[16]

The modification of ring A by the junction with a pyrazol ring or by the introduction of oxygen into position 2 considerably changes the conformation of ring A. This leads to an inconsistent increase of the anabolic activity. The introduction of alkyl substituents into ring A, in position C_1 (17β-hydroxy-1-methylandrost-1-en-3-one), C_2 (17β-hydroxy-2-methylandrost-1-en-3-one; 17β-hydroxy-2α-methylandrost-3-one), and C_7 (17β-hydroxy-7α,17α-dimethyl-androst-4-en-3-one) leads to intensified steroid anabolic activity. The removal of C_{19} methyl group considerably increases the anabolic effect and removes the steroid androgen action (ethyl-estrenol, 19-nortestosterone). The use of 19-testosterone was largely adopted for the synthesis of various AAS utilized in a clinical setting.

Thus, the discovery and consequent analysis of active androgen functional groups made it possible to create a rational basis for AAS-directed synthesis which found wide use in clinical medicine, endocrinology, and cattle breeding.

REFERENCES

1. **Duax, W. L. and Norton D.,** *Atlas of Steroid Structure,* Vol. I, Plenum Press, New York, 1975.
2. **Trager, L.,** *Steroidhormone, Biosynthese.* Stoffwechsel Wirkung, Berlin, 1977.
3. **Sergeev, P. V., Seifulla R. D., and Maisky, A. I.,** *Molecular Aspects of Steroid Hormones Action,* Nauka, Moscow, 1971.
4. **Kellie, A. E.,** Structure and nomenclature, in *Biochemistry of Steroid Hormones,* Makin, H. L. J., Ed., Blackwell Scientific Publications, Oxford, 1975, 1.
5. **Hall, E.,** The chemistry of the hormones, in *Hormone Analysis: Methodology and Clinical Interpretation,* Vol. I, Pennington, W. and Naik, S., Eds., CRC Press, Boca Raton, FL, 1981, 41.
6. **Duax, W. L., Weeks, C. M., and Rohier, D. C.,** Crystal structure of steroids: molecular conformation and biological function, *Rec. Prog. Horm. Res.,* 32, 81, 1976.
7. Revised Tentative Rules for Steroid Nomenclature IUPAC-IUB, 1967, Butterworth, London.
8. IUPAC Commission on Nomenclature of Organic Chemistry and IUPAC-IUB Commission on Biochemistry Nomenclature. Revised Tentative Rules for Nomenclature of Steroids, *Biochim. Biophys. Acta,* 164, 453, 1968.
9. IUPAC Commission on the Nomenclature of Organic Chemistry (CNOC) and IUPAC-IUB Commission on Biochemical Nomenclature (CBN) Amendments to Rules for Nomenclature of Steroids, *Biochem. J.,* 127, 613, 1972.
10. Steroid nomenclature, *J. Steroid Biochem.,* 21, 5, 1984.
11. Skeletal muscle pharmacology, Walter, W. G., Ed., *Excerpta Medica,* 1981, 188.
12. **Gower, D. B.,** Unsaturated C_{19} steroids. A review of their chemistry, biochemistry and possible physiological role, *J. Steroid Biochem.,* 3, 45, 1972.
13. **Gower, D. B. and Fortherly, K.,** Biosynthesis of the androgens and oestrogens, in *Biochemistry of Steroid Hormones,* Maken, H. L. J., Ed., Blackwell Sci. Publ., Oxford, 1975, 77.

14. **Liao, S., Liang, T., Fang, S., Castenada, E., and Shao, T.-C.,** Steroid structure and androgenic activity. Specificities involved in the receptor binding and nuclear retention of various androgens, *J. Biol. Chem.,* 248, 6154, 1973.
15. **Camerino, B. and Sciaky, R.,** Structure and effects of anabolic steroids, *Pharmacol. Ther.,* 1, 233, 1975.
16. **Pivnitsky, K.K.,** Anabolic steroid hormones, problems of testing and the bond of activities with structure, *Problems Endocrinol. USSR,* 4, III, 1974.
17. **Litvinova, V. N. and Rogozkin, V. A.,** Structure and metabolism of anabolic-androgenic steroids, in *Medicine and Sports,* Leningrad, 1979, 86.
18. **Dorfman, R. J. and Kincl, F. A.,** Relative potency of various steroids in an anabolic-androgenic assay using the castrated rat, *Endocrinology,* 72, 259, 1963.
19. **Arnold, A., Potts, G. O., and Beyler, A. L.,** Evaluation of the protein anabolic properties of certain orally active anabolic agents based on nitrogen balance studies in rats, *Endocrinology,* 72, 408, 1963.
20. **Kochakian, C. D.,** Renotrophic-androgenic properties of orally administrated androgens, *Proc. Soc. Exp. Biol.,* 80, 386, 1952.
21. **Scow, R. O. and Hagan, S. N.,** Effect of testosterone propionate on myosin, collagen and other protein fractions in striated muscles of gonadectomized male guinea pigs, *Am. J. Physiol.,* 180, 31, 1955.
22. **Kochakian, C. D. and Endhal, B. R.,** Influence of androgens on transaminase activities of different tissues, *Am. J. Physiol.,* 186, 460, 1956.
23. **Kochakian, C. D., Humm, J. H., and Bartlett, M. N.,** Effect of steroids on the body weight, temporal muscle and organs of the guinea pig, *Am. J. Physiol.,* 155, 242, 1948.
24. **Kochakian, C. D. and Tillotson, C.,** Influence of several C_{19} steroids on the growth of individual muscles of the guinea pig, *Endocrinology,* 60, 607, 1957.
25. **Sala, G. and Baldratti, G.,** A long-acting anabolic steroid: 4-hydroxy-19-nortestosterone-17-cyclopentylpropionate, *Endocrinology,* 72, 494, 1963.
26. **Nittling, E. F., Klinston, P. D., Gounsell, R. E., Overbeek, G. A., and de Visser, J.,** A comparison of the myotrophic and androgenic activities of the phenylpropionates and decanoates of testosterone and nandrolone, *Acta Endocrinol.,* 38, 285, 1961.
27. **Boris, A., Stevenson, R. H., and Trimol, T.,** Comparative androgenic, myotrophic and antigonadotrophic properties of some anabolic steroids, *Steroids,* 15, 61, 1970.
28. **Nutting, E. F., Klimstra, P. D., and Counsell, R. E.,** Anabolic-androgenic activity of A-ring modified androstene derivatives. I. Comparison of parenteral activity, *Acta Endocrinol.,* 53, 627, 1966.
29. **Nutting, E. F., Klimstra, P. D., and Counsell, R. E.,** Anabolic-androgenic activity of A-ring modified androstene derivatives. II. Comparison of oral activity, *Acta Endocrinol.,* 53, 635, 1966.
30. **Sommerwille, I. P. and Collins, W. P.,** Indices of androgen production in women, *Adv. Steroid Biochem. Pharmacol.,* 2, 266, 1970.
31. **Toth, M.,** Relative androgenic and myotrophic activity plots of 19-nortestosterone, *J. Steroid Biochem.,* 14, 1085, 1981.

Chapter 2

EXTRACELLULAR ANDROGEN BINDING PROTEINS

Before attempting an analysis of intracellular AAS metabolism, it is necessary to address a number of problems which are associated with hormone transport in the organism. It is an important starting point for realizing AAS action.

This group of steroid hormones, in physiological concentrations, has a pronounced effect on certain tissues and the capability to induce alterations of metabolic processes within them. The tissues or cells selectively responding to a steroid or some other hormones are usually called target tissues, or target cells, while other tissues are usually called hormone-resistant.[1] AAS possess a large spectrum of action which is manifested both in different kinds of tissues and in a variety of regulatory pathways in cells of the same type.

The trend, the duration, and the nature of metabolic effects caused by steroid hormones depend upon the structure of the hormone and phenotypical features of the target organs.

Each hormone, including AAS, selectively affects specific tissues in an organism and causes a metabolic alteration that allows an examination of the action as a specific hormonal effect. On the other hand, the variety of metabolic alterations and the heterogeneity of target tissues which leads to the multiplicity of the hormonal effect should be taken into account. Therefore, AAS may be considered to be a steroid hormone possessing a specific multiplicity of action.

In order to accomplish their function in an organism, AAS need to be delivered to the target organ. In every organism there exist the following kinds of proteins which are necessary for interaction with steroid hormones: transporter, receptor and enzymes. Each group of proteins accomplishes a certain function and is situated in certain organs and liquids.

AAS, like steroid hormones, are transported as complexes with binding proteins in the organism by blood. The binding of hormones in blood depends on their affinity for binding proteins and on the concentration of these proteins. With the binding of steroids, the proteins in the blood protect them against premature breakdown and against excessive quantities of free hormones in the blood. This results in a regulation of their concentration.

Androgens, estrogens, and AAS form complexes with testosterone-estradiol binding globulin (TEBG) in human blood. Several names are typically encountered in the literature: steroid binding β-globulin, globulin binding sexual hormones, steroid binding globulin and, more commonly, testosterone-estradiol binding globulin. Another transport protein, found in epididymis liquid, was named androgen binding protein (ABP). Hence, in organic fluids, there are two specific transport proteins which form dissociative complexes with AAS: TEBG in blood and ABP in epididymis fluid.

Additionally, the plasma albumin of blood, which binds low molecular substances, can bind steroids. Steroid hormones can appear in blood in three states: free, bound to TEBG, and bound to albumin. Though the affinity of TEBG for steroid hormones is 1000 times higher than that of albumin, the quantity of albumin in blood is 1000 times greater than that of TEBG. The binding index (the ratio of binding capability to the dissociation constant) of TEBG specific transport protein remains within the limits of the albumin binding index, and the steroid hormones can be equally distributed in blood between both binding proteins. Such a conclusion is confirmed by direct measurements of testosterone and the distribution of its active metabolite in blood. In men 45% of testosterone is bound to TEBG in blood, 53% is bound to albumin, and only 2% of testosterone is in a free state. In women these values are 62, 37 and 1% respectively.[2]

The basic transport protein in human blood is TEBG and appears to be glycoprotein with a carbohydrate content of 18 to 32% based on molecular weight. TEBG secreted from blood and liver cytoplasm has a molecular weight of 94,000 and consists of two subunits. The protein has one active center for steroid binding. While investigating the structural specificity of TEBG interaction with steroids, it was determined that the protein was capable of binding various steroids. This process depends on the presence of different functional groups and the topography of their position in the steroid molecule.[3] It was determined that the alteration of the functional group of 5α-position, the reduction Δ^4 of a double bond and the presence of 10β-methyl and 17α-ethyl groups improves the affinity for TEBG. To increase affinity for TEBG, a free 17β-OH group is also needed; however the 17β-oxy derivatives of steroids can interact with this transport protein. Still other modifications of the functional group, the presence of alkyl substituents in C_2, C_6, C_7, and C_{17} positions, as well as those of halogen in position C_2 or hydroxyl in position C_{11}, lead to a reduction in the affinity for TEBG.

In recent years we have witnessed the development of the concept in which the mechanism of TEBG interaction with steroid hormones consists of a steroid attraction to a TEBG active center by functional groups in positions C_3 and C_{17}. The active TEBG center has both similarities and differences to the active ABP center. This makes it possible to distinguish these transport proteins according to an interaction structural specificity with steroids.[3]

The funciton of TEBG in an organism is associated not only with AAS transport, but with their protection from breakdown during transport to target organs and regulation of the velocity of hormone migration to cells, thus affecting intracellular metabolism. In this way not only AAS themselves, but also their active metabolites, are subjected to binding to TEBG. TEBG synthesis occurs in the liver from which the protein migrates to the blood. The control for TEBG concentration in the blood may be carried out at the level of hormones. The rise of the concentration of estrogen and thyroid hormones increases the TEBG content in blood. On the contrary, decreasing the content of these hormones causes reduction of the binding protein concentration. It should be noted that there is little current experimental evidence on the metabolic behavior of TEBG, and many aspects of the behavior of this protein remain largely unknown.

The second specific transport protein (ABP) is found in epididymis and testis. ABP synthesis occurs in Sertoli cells and through tubular lumen protein and is secreted to the epididymis where it binds to androgens. ABP was isolated from the epididymis of a human being, a rabbit, and a rat. For a long time ABP was identified with TEBG since both proteins have similar physical and chemical properties, but they differ in their synthesis site. The use of highly selective purification methods, in particular column chromatography using concanavalin A, separates TEBG from ABP with a high degree of reliability.

The ABP isolated from human epididymis has a molecular weight of 90,000 and consists of two subunits. ABP is glycoprotein and in the presence of sialic acid can be broken down into a few glucose molecules and protein. The study of the specificity of various steroid APB binding sites revealed that in addition to testosterone and dihydrotestosterone, the protein bound strongly to androgen derivatives. A number of alterations in steroid structure have an essential influence on the affinity for ABP. It was shown that the reduction of Δ^4-double bond, 2α-alkyl groups, and the presence of 10β-methyl group usually improve steroid affinity for ABP. Other alterations in functional groups do not have such obvious effects on the affinity for ABP.[3]

The problem of hormonal control of ABP metabolism is still debatable. It has been established that multiple injection of testosterone-propionate into the organism intensifies ABP migration to epididymis. Concurrently, estrogen injections increase ABP androgen binding in sex tissues. The follicle-stimulating hormone increases the release of ABP into epididymis and blood. Testosterone has a stabilizing effect on ABP binding activity and this property can be used during protein isolation and purification.[4]

A number of TEBG and ABP physical-chemical properties are quite similar. The molecular weights of TEBG and ABP are 94,000 and 90,000, and the dissociation time constants with testosterone are 12.8 and 11 to 14 min, respectively. On the other hand, some alterations in the kinetics of ion exchange properties of DEAE (cellulose) were revealed in these proteins.[3]

Table 5 gives data showing the degree of various AAS and androgens binding to transport proteins. One can see that both proteins tightly bind separate hormones and their active metabolites. TEBG binds 5α-dihydrotestosterone most actively. The comparison of the various properties of these transport proteins enables us to note numerous coinciding indices that testify to their biological behavior. The different synthesis sites of these androgen binding transport proteins also determine the level of their participation in androgenic and AAS metabolism. While any target cell in the organism may be a site of action for TEBG, ABP action is restricted to the reproductive system. TEBG is synthesized in the liver and then migrates into blood and ensures steroid transport to target cells. The possibility of TEBG penetration into target organs slated for androgens was shown by means of immunochemical methods.[5] In the cells of

TABLE 5
Androgens and AAS Binding by
Extracellular Transport Proteins (%)

Steroid	TEBG	ABP
Testosterone	100	79
5α-Dihydrotestosterone	240	100
17β-Hydroxy-17α-methyl-androstan-3-one	65	74
19-Nortestosterone	18	—

target organs a steroid hormone may be bound to TEBG, androgen receptors, and enzyme systems participating in its metabolism. The amount of TEBG may influence the sensitivity of cells to androgen and change the velocity and intensity of the hormonal effect. It was shown that both free and bound protein androgens penetrate through the cellular membrane into liver with equal velocity. A high permeability of androgens to hepatocyte cellular membranes appears to be the primary factor for the rapid transport of hormones bound to protein. It should be taken into consideration that these substances have a high solubility in lipids, and the whole transport process through the membrane occurs without participation of specific carriers only owing to free diffusion. When studying the velocity of steroid transport to hepatocytes of liver and brain cells, lower values of hormone transport were found for the brain.[6]

While examining ABP functions it should be noted that the scale is considerably smaller. It is limited to sex tissues only. This protein ensures androgen transport and distribution only in the organs of the reproductive system.

A reversible binding to specific transport proteins circulating with AAS blood selectively restricts their migration to target organs. Various androgens, their active metabolites, and AAS compete for the transport protein binding sites. They are able to displace a familiar hormone from the complex with protein. In such conditions the concentration of a free hormone in blood increases and hence increases the possibility for its penetrating into the cell and its subsequent binding to cytoplasmic androgen receptors. Another way for regulating the level of androgen binding by blood transport proteins may be by androstenediols. Their synthesis occurs in prostate cells during the process of androgen metabolism. The androstenediols secreted from prostate to blood may displace testosterone and AAS from binding to TEBG. This results in increasing the concentration of free testosterone in blood which then migrates to a prostate cell, and under the action of the enzyme 5α-reductase, it converts to 5α-dihydrotestosterone. The latter is bound to cytoplasmic androgen receptors, and a new receptor cycle begins. This method of regulation includes transport proteins at one stage and ensures an adequate androgen concentration in the prostate.

Hence, a distinguishing feature of androgen binding transport proteins appears to be an active participation in the processes of androgens and AAS transport and their distribution among the organs as well as their control of metabolic processes which are associated with manifesting specific multiple hormonal effects.

REFERENCES

1. **Gorski, J., Toft, D., and Shyamala, L.**, Hormone-receptors: studies on interaction of estrogens with uteri, *Rec. Progr. Horm. Res.*, 24, 45, 1968.
2. **Södergard, R., Bäckstrom, T., Shanbhang, V., and Carstensen, H.**, Calculation of free and bound fractions of testosterone and estradiol-17β to human plasma proteins at body temperature, *J. Steroid Biochem.*, 16, 801, 1982.
3. **Lobt, T. J.**, Androgen transport proteins: physical properties, hormonal regulation and possible mechanism of TEBG and ABP action, *Arch. Androl.*, 7, 133, 1981.
4. **Tindall, D. J., Gunningham, G. R., and Means, A. R.**, 5α-Dihydrotestosterone binding to androgen binding protein, *J. Biol. Chem.*, 253, 166, 1979.
5. **Bardin, C. W., Musto, N., Gunsalus, G., Kotite, N., Cheng, S. L., Larrea, F., and Becker, R.**, Extracellular androgen binding proteins, *Annu. Rev. Physiol.*, 43, 189, 1981.
6. **Pardridge, W. M. and Mietus, L. J.**, Transport of protein-bound steroid hormones into liver in vivo, *Am. J. Physiol.*, 237, E367, 1979.
7. **Pugeat, M. M., Dunn, J. F., and Nisula, B. C.**, Transport of steroid hormones: interaction of 70 drugs with testosterone-binding globulin and corticosteroid-binding globulin in human plasma, *J. Clin. Endocrinol. Metab.*, 53, 69, 1981.

Chapter 3

AAS INTRACELLULAR RECEPTION

The ideas about the succession of events in the transmission of a hormone signal into the cell have recently been evolving. For steroid hormones this process is associated with the presence of a system of receptors inside the cell. The proteins that bind to a steroid hormone and deliver it to the place of active participation in cell metabolism appear to be the receptors of steroid hormones. A molecule of the receptor can be considered to be the first molecular element which recognizes a specific extracellular signal. Then, by means of a selective binding in the chain of intracellular reactions, a hormone response is formed.

All androgen receptors are found inside the cell and according to their location they can be divided into cytoplasmic and nuclear receptors. The experiments using AAS marked by tritium clearly showed the potential of these hormones in various tissues, primarily sex organs, liver, kidneys, skeletal muscles and heart. Over a long period of time either steroid or its active metabolite accumulates in these tissues.

In the process of studying these androgen receptors in animal tissues, some principal factors typical for their normal functioning in a cell were revealed. Among them one can note such properties of receptor as structural and steric specificity, limited capacity and saturation, hormone specificity and high affinity. A high velocity of receptor metabolism and their high modificative variability stipulated by the processes of phosphorylation, methylation and acetylation of receptor molecules was also revealed. It also was shown that receptors may be repeatedly used, which suggests the existence of a closed receptor cycle.

The most basic method of identification of androgen receptors is based on their capability to selectively, and their relative strength, bind to androgens and their metabolites. By analyzing the androgen-receptor interaction it becomes evident that this interaction is reversible and that the binding kinetics is determined by means of the law of active masses. During the hormone (S) and receptor (R) interaction, a hormone-receptor complex (SR) is formed.

$$S + R \xrightleftharpoons[K_{-1}]{K_{+1}} SR \tag{1}$$

where K_{+1} and K_{-1} are association and dissociation velocity constants of the hormone-receptor complex. The value K_{+1} is determined by the velocity with which S and R carry out the interaction and form an active hormone-receptor complex between each other. The value K_{-1} is inversely dependent on the strength of binding between steroid and receptor. As the hormone-receptor complex accumulates, the formation is retarded, while the dissociation is intensified. Then, after a certain period of time, a dynamic equilibrium is attained where the velocity of the hormone-receptor complex formation is equal to the velocity of its dissociation.

From the dissociation,

$$\frac{K_{+1}}{K_{-1}} = K_a = \frac{1}{K_d} = \frac{(SR)}{(S) \times (R)} \tag{2}$$

where K_a is an association or binding constant and K_d is a hormone-receptor complex dissociation constant. K_a defines the correlation between the bound steroids and the receptors which are free from the hormone under the conditions of equilibrium. The concentration of the hormone-receptor complex is in proportion to the constant of association, as well as to the concentration of steroid molecules and free receptors.

While studying the kinetic parameters of AAS and receptor interaction, there occurs the binding of a steroid molecule to one type of binding center of a receptor molecule. For this reason as a rule, K_a, K_d and N are determined as the concentration of receptor binding centers. To determine these values, one incubates a constant quantity of the receptor protein of interest with increasing concentrations of steroids marked by radioactive isotopes. After establishing an equilibrium, the fractions of free and bound steroids are divided and the content of the radioactivity in them is measured. The dependence of the hormone-receptor complex formation on steroid concentration is most often subjected to an analysis by drawing a Scatchard plot.[1]

For this reason the equation is transformed into the form

$$\frac{(SR)}{S} = K_a[N - (SR)] \tag{3}$$

or more conveniently

$$\frac{B}{U} = K_a(N - B) \tag{4}$$

where B is a bound hormone and U is an unbound hormone.

When plotting B/U versus B it becomes evident that there exists a linear dependence between the quantity ratio of bound and unbound steroid molecules to the concentration of hormone-receptor complex. When giving the data of a specific AAS binding in a Scatchard plot, the relationship is frequently linear, pointing out the homogeneity of binding sites.[2]

The plot represents a straight line with a slope that gives the value of N on the X-axis and the value K_a on the Y-axis. To determine the quantity of binding sites in a tissue one usually uses the value N and calculates milligrams of protein by taking into consideration the error of measuring the radioactivity, the volume of the sample, the quantity of protein and the value of B_{max}. As Figure 7 shows, the quantity of binding sites of androgen cytoplasmic receptors in rat skeletal muscles is $B_{max} = 0.6 \pm 0.2$ fmol/mg protein. [2]

The experiment shows that while investigating cytoplasmic and nuclear

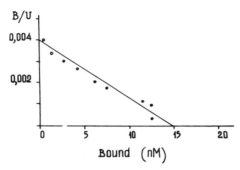

FIGURE 7. Scatchard analysis of ³H-19-nortestosterone binding by androgen receptors in rat skeletal muscle cytosol.

androgen receptors, two types of hormone and protein interactions occur: a non-specific interaction stipulated by the presence of ballast proteins (it is characterized by a low affinity and unlimited capacity) and a specific binding to receptor proteins based on a selective interaction with high affinity. To determine the level of nonspecific binding in the total quantity of androgen binding radioactivity, one usually adds 100 to 1000 units of unlabeled homrone.

A wide dispersion on the Scatchard plot for the experimental findings in the investigations on the interaction of various steroids with receptors is, to a certain degree, conditioned by a sufficient homogeneity of binding sites. However, it is possible to have several hormone-binding centers which differ in their affinity for the hormone. The Scatchard plot of such a binding is then represented as a curve which is concave in the direction of the bottom of the coordinates. In such cases other experimental findings may be used to form the plot.[3–5]

According to existing theories, the receptors in cells are in one of two states: free or bound to a hormone. By determining the receptor binding ability, one usually can determine a free receptor fraction unoccupied by the hormone. To measure the total quantity of receptors in a cell, it is necessary to release the occupied receptors from the hormone, that is to carry out a dissociation of existing hormone-receptor complexes. There are several methods for separating the hormone from its receptor, but unfortunately each of these methods has certain limitations. First, there is a rise of incubation temperature (up to 30) which not only causes the dissociation of hormone-receptor complexes, but also leads to an inactivation of the receptor as occurs in skeletal muscles. Second, the use of specific reagents accelerates the process of hormone-receptor complex dissociation.[6,7] Third, there is the use of the ligand interchange method.[8,9]

The first theory is based on the already established fact that the greatest accumulation of androgens occurs in ventral and dorsal prostate, as well as in seminal vesicles. Two to three hours after ³H-testosterone injection, the radioactivity in these tissues appears to be ³H-dihydrotestosterone which possesses a higher affinity for androgen receptors. Two proteins which actively bind hormone-receptor complexes with dihydrotestosterone, testosterone and AAS were revealed in prostate cytosol. The first, named β-protein, is precipitated by 20% saturated ammonia sulfate. It has a high affinity for dihydrotestosterone and 7α,17α-dimethyl-19-nortestosterone. The other receptor, α-protein, is precipitated by 55 to 70% saturated ammonia sulfate and tightly binds to testostertone, dihydrotestosterone and their metabolites. During extraction, using a solution 0.4 M KCl, both cytoplasmic androgen receptors have a sedimentation coefficient of about 3.5 S.[10] Only α-protein can form a hormone-receptor complex with dihydrotestosterone and testosterone and penetrate into the nucleus of a prostate cell. It was determined that α-protein has tissue specificity, since it was only found in cytoplasm and prostate nuclei. By using DNA-cellulose and the method of isoelectrofocusing, it was possible to purify the cytoplasmic androgen receptor from prostate 2000 times. In prostate cytoplasm, the number of binding sites for dihydrotestosterone is 100 fmol/mg protein or 4000 to 10,000 per cell. These values are twice that of other tissues, such as skeletal muscle and liver. The androgen receptors extracted from prostate nuclei, in solutions of a low ionic strength, are similar to cytoplasmic receptors when compared by their dimensions. The prostate nuclei can accumulate 200 to 6000 receptors per cellular nucleus. Ion-exchange analysis of cytoplasmic androgen receptors from hamster prostate on columns with DEAE-cellulose, DNA-cellulose and phosphocellulose made it possible to reveal their heterogeneity.[11] It was determined that a receptor functional form appears to be a dimer which consists of two subunits. The dimer has a sedimentation constant of 6 S while each subunit is 4 S. Such a dimer is supposed to be able to bind two moles of a steroid. Such a receptor consists of two functionally different parts. Subunit A contains a hormone-binding center and subunit B has a binding center with DNA. The active subunit A can express its function only through subunit B.

To elicit the structure of the androgen receptor binding center, the ability of a low molecular substance, similar in structure, to compete with a labeled androgen for binding to rat ventral prostate cytoplasmic receptor was investigated.[12] It was shown that the presence and order of the functional groups in steroid molecules are of great importance for the process of hormone binding to a receptor. It was determined that the selectivity of steroid binding to a receptor is defined mainly by 7α and 17α positions of hormone structure. The inclusion of methyl or other functional groups in these positions has a considerable effect on the degree of steroid-receptor affinity. Therefore, the interaction of 19-nortestosterone derivatives with the receptors greatly increases when the methyl group is present in 17α position. The methyl group in 7α position shows a much higher affinity. 7α,17α-Dimethyl-19-nortestosterone has an affinity for the receptor that can even exceed that of 5α-dihydrotestosterone. It has been suggested that the receptor contains a special local center (M-center) which interacts with 7α-methyl group. When the receptor interacts with a hormone, some conformational modifications in the protein molecule occur and this leads to a strong binding of these molecules. The plane of a steroid molecule is of greater importance in the interaction with the receptor that the electron structure of the ring-A bonds. This state may be observed in the example of converting testosterone to dihydrotestosterone under the action of the enzyme C_{19}-steroid-5α-reductase. In the course of the reaction not only will the removal of ring-A double bond in a testosterone molecule occur, but the structure of dihydro-testosterone changes too. It becomes flatter and interacts with the binding center of cytoplasmic prostate androgen receptor.[10] By investigating 60 different substances, which are similar to testosterone based on structure, only phenan-threne derivatives showed a strong specific binding to androgen receptor within the limits of concentrations from 20 mM to 2 mM. In the molecule of 9,10-dihydrophenanthrene two aromatic rings are bound to sites on the receptor molecule which are usually occupied by androgen rings B and D.[12]

The synthesis of 16β- and 16α-phenylselenotestosterone was described, and the investigation of their interaction with androgen receptors in various tissues was carried out. It was shown that these combinations have very low values of binding (0.1 to 0.3%), and this fact makes it difficult to obtain a reliable biological effect.[13]

The study of the affinity of androgen receptor ligands by means of various synthetic androgen and AAS makes it possible to not only realize the essence of the receptor process, but also to reveal a group specificity and plan the ways of further purposeful synthesis of new AAS and antihormones.

Understanding the mechanism of androgen receptor actions showing the existence of diverse molecular forms of receptors is of great importance. The use of centrifugation at the gradient of density and gel-filtration in media with low and high ionic strength revealed a complex quaternary structure of androgen receptors. The androgen receptors with a sedimentation coefficient of 8 to 9 S and a molecular mass of 200,000 to 300,000 daltons were revealed in the cytosol of various tissues in media with low ionic strength, their forms being asymmetric. By increasing the ionic strength to 0.15 M, the size of androgen receptor molecules diminishes. In these conditions the molecular mass of the receptors is 60,000 to 90,000 daltons and has sedimentation coefficients of 3.5 to 4.5 S.

The instability of 8 to 9 S molecules in physiological concentrations of salts led to a possible function of the large forms of receptors. However, a thorough analysis of such androgen receptor forms showed that it consisted of at least two proteins, a 4 to 5 S form (the androgen receptor itself) and a protein promoting the formation of 8 to 9 S form. The latter was subjected to a thorough purification and its molecular weight was 170,000.[14] The basic function of such a protein is associated with the formation of heavy assemblies during the interaction with 4 to 5 S receptor form. They appear to be 8 to 9 S androgen binding receptor forms. The protein was present in practically all tissues which are susceptible to androgens and which contain the androgen receptors. They include prostate, epididymis, testicle, spermatic vesicles, liver, thymus, kidneys, lungs, and heart.[14] The presence of this protein in blood serum may be the consequence of secretion from various androgen binding tissues. The rise of the concentration of this protein during the growth of the organism reflects the process of hormonal regulation.

By raising the ionic strength, or by changing the temperature, the sizes of androgen receptors diminish considerably and less aggregated forms of receptors with a sedimentation coefficient of 4 to 5 S appear. The existence of these two forms in dynamic equilibrium is quite possible. It was confirmed by two-phase saturation and by the presence of two centers of androgen binding to be equal to K_d. The findings of these investigations, the physical and chemical properties of androgen receptor complexes formed in rat prostates during experiments *in vivo* and *in vitro*, showed that the values K_d for dihydrotestosterone and methyltrienolone in both cases make up 0.3 nM.[15] It demonstrates a considerable alliance of dissociation velocities of such hormone-receptor complexes. At the same time, the analysis of separate properties of these androgen receptor complexes revealed considerable differences in the measurements *in vivo* and *in vitro*. First of all, they are concerned with common indices such as the molecular weight of the complex, which as determined according to a sedimentation constant for the androgen receptor complex was 7 to 8 S, while in the experiments *in vivo* the value for the same complex was lower — 5 to 6 S. The use of mersalic acid as a chemical agent, which interacts with SH-groups of receptors and accelerates the dissociation of hormone-receptor complexes, proved to be sufficiently effective only in the experiments *in vitro*.[7] In the experiments *in vivo*, mersalic acid had little effect on the dissociation of the hormone-receptor complex. These factors show that conformational modifications in a receptor molecule by interacting with a hormone *in vivo* are considerably different from those in the experiments *in vitro*. When comparing these and some other factors characterizing the formation of androgen-receptor complex, one may draw a conclusion as to the considerable alteration of complex affinities which are formed in rat prostate *in vivo*. Such differences are stipulated by profound conformational modifications of a receptor molecule and cannot be completely reproduced in *in vitro* experiments. Some limitations in the use of mersalic acid to determine the receptors occupied by androgens are clearly shown. The release of the receptors from hormones under the action of mersalic acid occurs only in the experiments *in vitro*.[15]

For many years the attention of investigators studying the mechanism of androgen action in organisms was basically attracted to the organs of the sex system, where an androgen influence was being most distinctly revealed. Some attempts in determining the possibility of androgen binding in other tissues have been unsuccessful in recent times because of poor methods, low affinity and a small number of androgen receptors. One theory suggested that skeletal and cardiac muscles have no special receptor apparatus for androgen binding. In his monograph published in 1977, one of the most prominent specialists on the mechanism of androgen action denied the presence of special androgen receptors in skeletal muscles.[16] It was suggested that if the mechanism of androgen binding in skeletal muscles does not exist, it absolutely differs by its nature from that of prostate.[17-19] To prove it scientifically, one cites some findings on a high lability and a small number of receptors, as well as the differences between androgen binding sites and anabolic ones in muscular tissue.[20] By a more thorough examination of the first works concerning the study of AAS binding in muscles, some investigations of Mayer and Rosen could be noted.[21] These authors were not able to show specific androgen receptors in skeletal muscle, but they established that AAS (methyltestosterone, methandrostenolone, nandrolone, fluoxymesterone and others) could interact with glucocorticoid receptors in skeletal muscle cytosol and this process led to decreasing dexamethasone and cortisol binding. According to the results, 2 hours after a single AAS injection a decrease in glucocorticoid binding in cytoplasm of muscular tissue was observed. Such AAS as norethandrolone and fluoxymesterone compete most strongly for glucocorticoid binding sites in cytosol. A prolonged AAS use (4 injections for 4 days) also showed that these hormones had the ability to sharply suppress glucocorticoid binding in skeletal muscles. These results led the authors to conclude that the androgens possess an antiglucocorticoidal action in skeletal muscle cytosol. Unfortunately, although this investigation shows the possibility of AAS binding in muscular tissue, we do not have sufficient knowledge about the question of which receptors AAS do interact with. From these results we tried to solve two problems in a number of experiments. First, we estimated the possibility of binding one of the most widespread AAS, nandrolone-decanoate, in skeletal muscles in the presence of testosterone, and second, we attempted to demonstrate the possibility of a competition between AAS and glucocorticoids for binding sites in muscle tissue. The findings of these investigations are given in Table 6 and in Figure 8.

It turned out that after injecting nandrolone-decanoate into an organism, ^{3}H-testosterone binding in skeletal muscles radically decreased (to 33%). The decrease of testosterone binding to transport protein was also marked. From the results it was concluded that testosterone and nandrolone-decanoate compete in skeletal muscles for common androgen receptors.

While investigating a competitive 19-nortestosterone and glucocorticoid binding it was shown (Figure 8) that dexamethasone and corticosterone had no

TABLE 6
The Effect of Nandrolone-Decanoate on
^{3}H-Testosterone Including in Rat Skeletal Muscles

Experimental conditions	Radioactivity of skeletal muscles (dpm/mg tissue)	Blood radioactivity (dpm/ml)
Without hormone	160 5	270 6
With nandrolone-decanoate	106 9	246 9

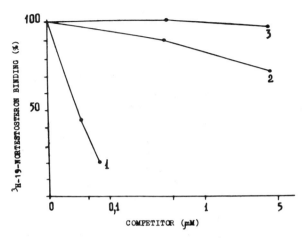

FIGURE 8.   Competition of glucocorticoids with ³H-19-nortestoster-
one for specific binding to the rat muscle androgen receptor. 19-
Nortestosterone, 1; dexamethasone, 2; corticosterone, 3.

effect on the AAS interaction with the receptor. Hence, AAS are effectively
bound by androgens and not by glucocorticoid receptors in skeletal muscle.
Subsequent investigations confirmed the results on the differences in physical-
chemical properties of androgen receptors and glucocorticoids in skeletal
muscles.[22] It took some years of serious methodical work, years which considerably improved the study of hormone-receptor interaction, before the presence
of androgen receptor in numerous tissues became quite obvious.

In recent years, the development of techniques employed in steroid hormone
receptor experiments has helped to ascertain the presence of cytoplasmic
androgen receptors in skeletal and cardiac muscles.[23–29]

A high thermolability of androgen hormone-receptor complexes in skeletal
muscles creates considerable complications in obtaining reliable data on a
number of receptors. The rise of temperature in an incubation process rapidly
leads to a receptor inactivation and makes it difficult to reliably determine the
number of free and occupied hormone androgen receptor binding sites. In order
to avoid the rapid loss in the binding ability of cytoplasmic proteins in skeletal
muscle, an attempt to stabilize such proteins was made. It became necessary to
search for substances that would be able to have a stabilizing effect on receptor
molecules. The hormone itself, the protectors of SH-groups, glycerine and
molybdate ions possess a stabilizing effect on androgen binding sites of the
receptor molecule. The study of the kinetics of the association and dissociation
of androgen-receptor complexes showed that all these substances may retain
binding properties of androgen receptors to some extent. The analysis of the
effect of various sulfhydryl chemical agents on receptor binding properties
revealed that active participation of SH-group protectors (dithiothreitol, mercap-

toethanol) in small concentrations led to some increase in androgen receptor binding properties, as well as to a stabilization of the receptor molecule.

Among various stabilizing factors affecting the cytoplasmic androgen receptors it is necessary to note (and it would not be an exaggeration) the important role of molybdate ions. Numerous investigations have clearly shown that the values of androgen binding in cytosol of various tissues in the presence of molybdate grew considerably.[30-32]

The ion of molybdate has a stabilizing effect on androgen receptors in a wide range of temperatures in a considerably narrow zone of pH. Sodium molybdate has no effect on the dissociation velocity of hormone with a receptor, but it increases the dissociation velocity of hormone-receptor complex. The mechanism of the stabilizing effect of molybdate ions on androgen receptors may be associated with:

1. Stabilization of phosphate groups of receptor molecules which decreases its affinity for proteolytic enzymes
2. Interaction with SH-groups of a receptor
3. Endogenetic phosphatase and ribonuclease inhibition, and
4. Inhibition of the dissociation of receptor oligomerous forms.

Therefore, the absence of an appreciable ion molybdate effect on the velocity of the initial interaction with a receptor and the retaining of a high receptor stability makes it possible to use molybdate ions in the investigations of various properties of androgen receptors.[33,34]

By studying AAS binding to androgen receptors in the cytoplasm of the skeletal muscle of rats (for isolating hormone-receptor complexes), some principal methods of protein fractionation are used: centrifugation in the gradient of a saccharose density, precipitation by ammonia sulfate salts and adsorption on coal covered with dextrane. In the last years ^{3}H-methyltrienolone (17β-hydroxy-17α-methylestra-4,9,11-trien-3-one) has been used as a labeled ligand. It has a high affinity for androgen receptors, and it is not subjected to metabolic conversions in the organism.[35,36]

One of the first muscles in which androgen receptors were revealed, with a certain reliability, was m.l.a. It turned out that this muscle contains much more androgen receptor than some other skeletal muscles, but the values are considerably less than in basic androgen-dependent tissues (e.g., ventral prostate). When using ^{3}H-methyltrienolone for determining androgen receptors in m.l.a., it was shown that the number of binding sites made up 8 fmol/mg of protein, and K_d was 0.74 nM.[37] Cytoplasmic androgen receptors from this muscle have the same kinetic characteristics and physical-chemical properties as do androgen receptors in other tissues. A comparative study of binding and metabolism of testosterone, dihydrotestosterone and 19-nortestosterone in prostate, m.l.a. and rat skeletal muscles showed that the basic physical-chemical characteristics of binding proteins in these tissues were similar, if not identical. Therefore, in muscles, they can also be called androgen receptors.[38] Some essential differences in the number of androgen binding sites were revealed. This value makes up 140 fmol/mg of protein in prostate, 24 fmol/mg of protein in m.l.a., and 2 fmol/mg of protein in skeletal muscles. A thorough study of 5α-reductase activity and the specificity of androgen binding protein in three tissues revealed a positive correlation between androgen action at the cell level and the number of binding sites, as well as between the activity of the enzyme 5α-reductase and the degree of receptor affinity for various androgens and their metabolites.[38]

Table 7 gives the K_d values and the content of binding sites of cytoplasmic androgen receptors in skeletal muscles of different animals.

One can see that the mean values of K_d are within the limits of 0.2 to 2.0 nM, and the concentration of binding sites of cytoplasmic receptors makes up 0.6 to 5.7 fmol/mg of protein.

The determination of the number of binding sites of cytoplasmic androgen receptors in rat skeletal muscle of both sexes and at different ages established the change of this index in the process of organism development.[22] Cytoplasmic androgen receptors in female skeletal muscles have lower values of K_d, but females have a higher number of binding sites in comparison with males.

After an animal was castrated, the differences in androgen reception efficiency in skeletal muscles were lost.

As the organism develops and its weight increases, a reduction in the number of androgen receptor binding sites in skeletal muscles is observed. Such AAS as stanosolol, 19-nortestosterone and 19-nortestosterone-decanoate effectively compete with testosterone and dihydrotestosterone for binding to androgen receptors in cytoplasm of skeletal muscles. The binding ability of androgen receptors and other parameters in the formation of cytoplasmic hormone-receptor complexes in mouse skeletal muscle with hereditary muscular dystrophy did not differ from the values obtained in healthy animals. One may conclude

TABLE 7
Androgen Receptors in
Mammalian Skeletal Muscle Cytosol

Subject	K_d (nM)	B_{max} (fmol/mg protein)	Ref.
Mouse	0.66	2.91	15
	0.60	2.80	26
Rat	0.19	3.10	15
	0.39	0.60	27
Human	0.28	1.1	18
Monkey heart	2.0	5.30	28
Mice with hereditary	0.44	2.77	15
muscular dystrophy	0.80	5.70	26

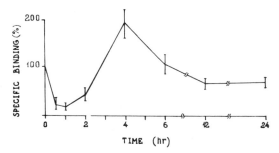

FIGURE 9. 19-Nortestosterone binding in rat skeletal muscle cytosol.

that clinical and functional symptoms of hereditary muscular dystrophy are not associated directly with the change in accumulation and the biological effect of androgens in muscles.[39]

The investigations carried out in the Gustaffson laboratory proved the presence of androgen receptors in cytosol of human skeletal muscles.[29] By determining the competition for binding sites, it was shown that 7α-methyl-19-nortestosterone was more active that 19-nortestosterone and testosterone. K_d was 0.28×10^{-9} M of androgen receptors and the number of binding sites (1.1 to 4.0 fmol/mg of protein) was determined.

It was also established in this work that the content of androgen receptors in cytosol of female skeletal muscle is higher than that in males. It is probably associated with a high content of androgens in men which leads to a greater occupation of steroid receptors by endogenetic hormones.

Therefore, the human skeletal muscles have specific androgen receptors, and this tissue can directly respond to the presence of androgens in AAS.

The interaction of AAS with androgen receptors, as well as subsequent events stipulated by the formation and the migration of the hormone-receptor complex, are of essential significance for realizing the mechanism of action of AAS in the cell.

The results from this laboratory show that after a single injection of 19-nortestosterone into white rats, an appreciable alteration in the content of androgen receptors was observed in skeletal muscle cytosol (Figure 9).

As shown in Figure 9 after injecting a hormone into an animal, the number of free cytoplasmic androgen receptors rapidly decreases and in 30 to 60 minutes it is only 15 to 20% of the initial level. These alterations in the content of free androgen receptors are associated with the formation of hormone-receptor complexes due to the appearance of 19-nortestosterone molecules in cytoplasm and a further translocation of these complexes to the muscular cell nucleus. Two hours after injecting 19-nortestosterone, a gradual increase of AAS receptor binding in cytoplasm occurs and reaches maximum values by the fourth hour. The rise in the number of free cytoplasmic androgen receptors during 2 to 4 hours is associated with the migration of the receptors from the nucleus back into cytoplasm. Such conclusion is based on the measured values of 19-nortestosterone binding by nuclei from skeletal muscle, which was at maximum 2 hours after the hormone injection.

Hence, a single injection of 19-nortestosterone into an organism leads to the change in the number of free androgen receptors in skeletal muscle cytoplasm with the formation of a hormone-receptor complex and with its further translocation to a cellular nucleus.

By comparing the degree of affinity of various AAS for androgen receptors in skeletal muscle cytoplasm it was shown that 19-nortestosterone is bound to the receptor three times more strongly than testosterone is. The absence of the enzyme 5α-reductase in skeletal muscle leads to the rise in myotrophic activity in a series of AAS, primarily 19-nortestosterone and its derivatives.

The question of the synthesis of androgen receptors in skeletal muscles has not yet been tested experimentally. Measuring androgen binding in m.l.a. during the regenerating processes after a mechanical muscle injury could be a potential solution. It has been shown that on the second to third day after an injury, there is a sharp reduction in the content of androgen receptors. It is associated with the removal of the cytoplasm as well as with the restoration and the proliferation of myoblastic cell population.[37] The seventh day after the injury there was a growth in androgen binding and the restoration of receptor activity up to the initial values that occur during myoblast merging and the differentiation of myotubules to multinuclear, cross-stripped myofibrils. Thus, it is shown that the restoration of androgen binding in a muscle is closely associated with the presence of certain cellular structures and normal metabolism. This is the first investigation on the process of androgen-receptor development in skeletal muscle.

The investigations were carried out in a very convenient pattern. Mouse line Tfm, with full testicular feminization, showed that in the cells of a number of target organs, androgen receptors were absent or their activity was considerably reduced and made up 10 to 30% of the binding shown in healthy animals.[28]

Besides cytoplasmic androgen receptors, estrogen receptors were also found in the skeletal muscles of white rats.[42] It has been established that in the cytosol of skeletal muscle, there are receptor proteins which actively bind estradiol-17β where K_d makes up from 0.1 to 1.0 nM and it does not depend on temperature. B_{max} for estradiol-17β in cytosol of skeletal muscles makes up 120 fmol/mg of protein. A binding specifity for various synthetic hormones was also shown.

At present, many experimental findings showing the presence of androgen receptors in many tissues have been accumulated. Along with classical androgen-dependent tissues (testicle, prostate, adrenal, kidneys), androgen receptors were also found in tissues that formerly were thought to be androgen-resistant — liver, thymus, brain, skeletal and cardiac muscles.[29,41,43–45]

Numerous investigations have shown (and today it is beyond any doubt) the presence of a positive interaction between the values of hormone affinity for a receptor and biological hormone activity.

A certain threshold level of the intensity for ligand binding to a receptor is needed for manifesting the hormone effect.

One can believe that the hormone bound to a receptor with a sufficiently high K_a would cause conformational modifications in the receptor protein leading to the possibility of a subsequent manifestation of biological activity of the complex. The value K_a is one of the factors determining the effectiveness of formation of the complex. The threshold level K_a, where a ligand-receptor complex becomes effective for androgen receptors, makes up the value $10^7 M^{-1}$. It should be noted that the hormone bound by a receptor is protected against the action of enzymes; therefore the androgen binding protects them from inactivation. The discovery of molecular mechanisms of the hormone-receptor interaction is of great significance for revealing the process of hormone regulation in the cell. The possibility of a specific hormone binding to a receptor is dependent on size, stereostructure, and diffusive and electronic properties of the steroid molecules ensuring the steroid correspondence with a receptor binding center.[12]

Hence, in the cytoplasm of various tissues, there are a group of receptor proteins which selectively interact with androgens and AAS. The process of hormone-receptor interaction has a reversible character. It may be represented by a number of kinetic parameters. The concentration of binding sites of cytoplasmic androgen receptors has a limited capacity and makes up only 2 to 4 fmol/mg of protein. One of the most important characteristics of cytoplasmic androgen receptor binding sites is a stereospecificity of their affinity for certain hormones, that is the ability of receptors to selectively bind separate androgens, active metabolites and AAS, so that the androgen receptor of the prostate has a higher affinity for dihydrotestosterone than for testosterone. For the translocation of a cytoplasmic hormone-receptor complex to a nucleus, an activation of this complex, or its conversion to a form in which it is able to be bound to structural components of cell nuclei, is needed.

A few trends of influence, such as a rise in temperature and an increase in ionic strength, are possible. They lead to the activation of a hormone-receptor complex and its transformation into a lower molecular form thus allowing migration to a nucleus and specific interaction with chromatin. There is no strong evidence to indicate whether the activation includes an enzymatic modification or only includes conformational modifications in the hormone-receptor complex. However the transformation of the specific steroid-receptor complex into a form ensuring a further hormone signal transmission is supposed to take place here.

REFERENCES

1. **Scatchard C.**, The attraction of proteins for small molecules and ions, *Ann N.Y. Acad Sci.,* 51, 660, 1959.
2. **Rogozkin, V. A., Felskoren, B. I., Osipova, E. I., and Stepanov, M. G.,** Cytoplasmic and nuclear androgen receptor in skeletal muscle, in 16th Meet. FEBS, Moscow, June 1984, Abstr. 421.
3. **Rosenthal, H. E.,** A graphic method for the determination and presentation of binding parameters to a complex system, *Anal. Biochem.,* 20, 525, 1967.
4. **Munson, P. S. and Rodbard, D.,** Ligand, a versatile computerized approach for characterization of ligand-binding systems, *Anal. Biochem.,* 107, 220, 1980.
5. **Klotz, I. M.,** Numbers of receptor sites from Scatchard graphs: facts and fantasies, *Science,* 217, 1247, 1982.
6. **Sica, V., Puca, A., Molinari, A. M., Buonaguro, F. M., and Bresciani, F.,** Effect of chemical perturbation with NASCN on receptor-estradiol interaction, *Biochemistry,* 19, 83, 1980.
7. **Traish, A. M., Müller, R. E., and Wotiz, H. H.,** A new procedure for quantitative nuclear and cytoplasmic androgen receptors, *J. Biol. Chem.,* 256, 12026, 1981.
8. **Anderson, J., Clark, J., and Peck, J., Jr.,** Oestrogen and nuclear binding sites. Determination of specific sites by ^{3}H-oestradiol exchange, *Biochem. J.,* 126, 561, 1972.
9. **Hechter, O., Mechaber, D., Zwick, A., Camfield, L. A., Eychenne, B., Baulieu, E. E., and Robel, P.,** Optimal radioligand exchange conditions for measurement of occupied androgen receptor sites in rat ventral prostate, *Arch. Biochem. Biophys.,* 224, 49, 1983.
10. **Liao, S., Liang, T., Fang, S., Castaneda, E., and Shao, T.,** Steroid structure and androgen activity, *J. Biol. Chem.,* 248, 6154, 1973.
11. **Schrader, W. T., Selenzev, Y., Vedeckis, W. V., and O'Malley, B. W.,** Steroid receptor subunit structure, in *Gene Regulation by Steroid Hormones,* Roy, A. K. and Clark, J. H., Eds., Springer-Verlag, New York, 1980, 78.
12. **Liao, Sh., Chang, Ch., and Saltzman, A. G.,** Androgen-receptor interaction, in *Steroid Hormone Receptors: Structure and Function,* Friksson, A. and Gustafsson, A., Eds., Elsevier Science, Amsterdam, 1983, 407.
13. **Konopelski, J. P., Djerassi, C., and Raynaub, J. P.,** Synthesis and biochemical screening of phenylselenium-substituted steroid hormones, *J. Med. Chem.,* 23, 722, 1980.
14. **Colvard, D. S. and Wilson, E. M.,** Identification of an 8 S androgen receptor-promoting factor that converts the 4.5 S form of the androgen receptor to 8 S, *Endocrinology,* 109, 496, 1981.
15. **Traish, A. M., Müller, R. E., and Wotiz, H. H.,** Differences in the physicochemical characteristics of androgen-receptor complexes formed in vivo and in vitro, *Endocrinology,* 114, 1761, 1984.
16. **Mainwaring, W. I. P.,** *The Mechanism of Action of Androgens,* Springer-Verlag, New York, 1977.
17. **Ritzen, F. M., Nayfey, S. N., French, F. S., and Dobbins, M. L.,** Demonstration of androgen-binding components in rat epididymis cytosol and comparison with binding components in prostate and other tissues, *Endocrinology,* 89, 143, 1971.
18. **Mainwaring, W. I. P. and Mangan, F. R.,** A study of the androgen receptors in a variety of androgen-sensitive tissue, *J. Endocrinol.,* 59, 121, 1973.
19. **Krieg, M., Szalay, R., and Voigt, K. D.,** Binding and metabolism of testosterone and of 5α-dihydrotestosterone in bulboca-vernousus-levator ani (Bcla) of male rats: in vivo and in vitro studies, *J. Steroid Biochem.,* 5, 453, 1974.
20. **Steinitz, B. G., Grannini, T., Butler, M., and Popick, A.,** Dissociation of anabolic and androgenic properties of steroid by anti-anabolic and anti-androgenic agents in rats, *Endocrinology,* 89, 894, 1971.
21. **Mayer, M. and Rosen, F.,** Interaction of anabolic steroids with glucocorticoid receptor sites in rat muscle cytosol, *Am. J. Physiol.,* 225, 1381, 1975.

22. **Dahlberg, E., Snochowski, M., and Gustafsson, J. A.,** Regulation of the androgen and glucocorticoid receptors in rat and mouse skeletal muscle cytosol, *Endocrinology,* 108, 1431, 1981.
23. **Michel, G. and Baulieu, E. E.,** Androgen receptor in skeletal muscle, *J. Endocrinol.,* 65, 31P, 1975.
24. **Dube, J. Y., Lesage, R., and Tremblay, R. R.,** Androgen and estrogen binding in rat skeletal and perineal muscles, *Can. J. Biochem.,* 54, 50, 1976.
25. **Krieg, M.,** Characterization of the androgen receptor in the skeletal muscle of the rat, *Steroids,* 28, 261, 1976.
26. **Tremblay, R. R., Dube, J. Y., Ho-Kim, M. A., and Lesage, R.,** Determination of rat muscles androgen-receptor complexes with methyltrienolone, *Steroids,* 29, 185, 1977.
27. **Michel, G. and Baulieu, E. E.,** Androgen receptor in rat skeletal muscle: characterization and physiological variations, *Endocrinology,* 107, 2088, 1980.
28. **Max, S. R.,** Cytosolic androgen receptor in skeletal muscle from normal and testicular feminization mutant (Tfm) rats, *Biochem. Biophys. Res. Commun.,* 101, 792, 1981.
29. **Snochowski, M., Saartok, T., Dahlberg, E., Erikson, E., and Gustafsson, J.,** Androgen and glucocorticoid receptors in human skeletal muscle cytosol, *J. Steroid Biochem.,* 14, 765, 1981.
30. **Wright, W. W., Chan, K. C., and Bardin, C. W.,** Characterization of the stabilizing effect of sodium molybdate on the androgen receptor present in mouse kidney, *Endocrinology,* 108, 2210, 1981.
31. **Braun, B. E., Krieg, M., and Smith, K.,** Sexual environment and molybdate: two factors influencing on the androgen-receptor quantification in prostable, bulbocavernousus/levator ani and heart muscle of male Wistar rats, *Mol. Cell. Endocrinol.,* 26, 177, 1982.
32. **Sherman, M. R., Moran, M. C., Tuazon, F. B., and Yee-Won Stevens,** Structure dissociation and proteolysis of mammalian steroid receptors, *J. Biol. Chem.,* 258, 10336, 1983.
33. **Naritoku, W. Y., Howard, E. B., Britt, J. O., and Markland, F. S.,** Effect of molybdate on androgen receptor levels in canine prostate, *Prostate,* 3, 611, 1982.
34. **Dahmer, M. K., Housley, P. R., and Pratt, W. B.,** Effect of molybdate and endrogenous inhibitors on steroid-receptor inactivation, transformation and translocation, *Annu. Rev. Physiol.,* 46, 67, 1984.
35. **Bonne, C. and Raynand, J. P.,** Methyltrienolone, a specific ligand for cellular androgen receptor, *Steroids,* 26, 227, 1975.
36. **Bonne, C. and Raynand, J. P.,** Assay of androgen binding sites by exchange with methyltrienolone (R 1881), *Steroids,* 27, 497, 1976.
37. **Max, S. R., Mufti, S., and Carlson, B. M.,** Cytosolic androgen receptor in regenerating rat levator muscle, *Biochem. J.,* 200, 77, 1981.
38. **Krieg, M. and Voigt, K. D.,** In vitro binding and metabolism of androgens in various organs: a comparative study, *J. Steroid Biochem.,* 7, 1005, 1976.
39. **Max, S. R.,** Cytosolic androgen receptor in skeletal muscle from normal and dystrophic mice, *J. Steroid Biochem.,* 18, 281, 1983.
40. **Osipova, E. I. and Feldkoren, B. I.,** Determination of cytoplasmic receptors of androgens in skeletal muscles of intact albino rats, *Acta Commun. Univ. Tartuensis Tartu,* 679, 127, 1984.
41. **McGill, H. C., Anselmo, V. C., Buchanan, J. M., and Sherdian, P. J.,** The heart is a target organ for androgen, *Science,* 207, 775, 1980.
42. **Dahbberg, E.,** Characterization of the cytosol estrogen receptor in rat skeletal muscle, *Biochim. Biophys. Acta,* 717, 65, 1982.
43. **Tremblay, R. R., No-Kim, M. A., and Dube, J. Y.,** Characterization partielle et variations du recepteur cytoplasmique des androgenes dans le rein de rat, *Ann. Endocrinol.,* 44, 247, 1983.
44. **McGinnis M. Y., Davis, P. G., Meaney, M. J., Singer, M., and McEwen, B.,** In vitro measurement of cytosol and cell nuclear androgen receptors in male rat brain and pituitary, *Brain Res.,* 275, 75, 1983.

45. **Hickson, R., Galessi, T., Kurowski, T., Daniels, D., and Chatterton, R.,** Skeletal muscle cytosol ^{3}H-methyltrienolone receptor binding and serum androgens: effects of hypertrophy and hormonal state, *J. Steroid Biochem.,* 19, 1705, 1983.

Chapter 4

TRANSLOCATION OF CYTOPLASMIC HORMONE-RECEPTOR COMPLEXES TO CELLULAR NUCLEUS

The translocation of a hormone-receptor complex from cytosol to nuclei under the influence of hormones appears to be a general property of steroid hormone receptors; this property seems to be common for all the target organs and hormones. The principal biological significance of the translocation process is the fact that the interaction between the steroid-receptor complex and chromatin causes a modification of gene transcription and leads to the synthesis of hormone controlled proteins. The properties of the receptor are changed by steroid binding in such a way that it gains affinity for the nuclei. These alterations in a receptor molecule are called "activation". The hormone binding to a receptor and the hormone activation are not simultaneous, but rather successive events. It may be demonstrated by the fact that if target cells are incubated with a steroid at a low temperature, a steroid-receptor complex is formed in cytoplasm, and it remains here for a relatively long period of time before it is bound to nuclei. Under the influence of high temperatures, the complex develops the ability to interact with cellular nucleic membranes and may be translocated from cytoplasm to nucleus.

When hormonal information passes to the nucleus, the receptor may appear in at least two states: inactive and active.

When studying hormone-receptor complexes, the alteration of a receptor molecule structure was demonstrated. Although they were assigned the terms "activation" and "transformation", they are often used in the same sense. There also exists the possibility of differentiating these notions and connecting them with certain receptor physical-chemical properties. The term "transformation" of a receptor is tightly associated with the alterations of a molecular mass and the receptor molecular sizes that may be determined from different methods (sedimentation constant, the velocity of migration during electrophoresis or by electrofocusing). The term "activation" of a receptor can be defined as a conformational modification of receptor structure that leads to the appearance of the ability to bind to cellular nucleic components, primarily to chromatin. It appears to be an indispensable stage of cytoplasmic hormone-receptor complex translocation to cell nucleus.

A theoretical analysis of the possible mechanisms of receptor activation with regard to kinetic and thermodynamic information allows (and there are good reasons for this) the examination of two probable mechanisms. The first one includes a receptor dimerization and its interaction with an unknown molecule which occurs similarly to the reaction of the second order.[1] In this case the presence of one more molecules is needed. It was hypothesized that this is an activator of the activation which forms a complex with the receptor. Some attempts were made to explain, with the help of such a mechanism, temperature transformation of cytoplasmic estrogen receptors from 4 S form to 5 S form.[2] The second mechanism includes a simple conformational modification of a receptor molecule stipulated by the breaking of some noncovalent bonds without a direct interaction with a molecule of another substance. According to the kinetic parameters, such a reaction refers to the first order reaction.[3] Thus, the principal difference between the two mechanisms of receptor activation consists of the presence (the first variant) or the absence (the second variant) of another substance (except a hormone) which interacts with a receptor and causes its activation. Numerous investigations relating to the discovery of the mechanism of receptor activation were examined in detail in the literature.[2] It gives well-grounded kinetic results and thermodynamic calculations in favor of the mechanism of activation which assumes a conformational modification of receptor molecules.

The study of the mechanism of cytoplasmic androgen receptor activation showed that this effect may be obtained with the help of various influences. The most widespread method which is used for the activation of cytoplasmic androgen receptors and other steroid hormones is the incubation of patterns *in vitro* in the presence of ^{3}H-steroids at high temperature. The heating of cytosol containing androgen receptors in the presence of ^{3}H-hormone leads to the ability of a receptor to be translocated to nuclei and strongly bound to chromatin.

In experiments *in vitro*, in low ionic strength, physiological meaning and low temperature, receptor activation and the formation of hormone-receptor complexes occur extremely slowly. With an increase in temperature, the velocity of receptor-molecule activation sharply accelerates. This illustrates the point that the presence of a high energetic barrier, which should be overcome by the receptor molecule in order to turn into an active form, allows the interaction with hormone molecules. The energy of activation for the present process makes up 31 kcal, thus making some calculations possible as to the number of noncovalent bonds broken in the course of the activation.[3] If there are only hydrogenous and ionic bonds that are broken, then, assuming the energy of this bond to be equal to ~5 kcal, their quantity will make up 6 to 7 units. When only hydrophobic bonds with a lower bond energy participate in the activation process, the number of broken bonds becomes greater. The fact that the increase in incubation ionic strength accelerates the receptor activation and leads to a decrease in activation energy is rather important.

It is therefore apparent that in this case some bonds are broken and some conformational changes in the receptor molecule take place. It involves the ionic bonds which can be considerably weakened during the increase in ionic strength. The decrease of the activation of energy in the range of 0.05 to 0.4 M KCl shows that more than three ionic bonds are included in conformational changes of the receptor molecule. The fact that by increasing pH to 8 the reaction of receptor activation proceeds at 0° shows the possibility of the participation of one or a few positive charged groups with pK 6 to 8 in the formation of ionic bridges which stabilize the receptor molecule.

Activation of cytoplasmic androgen receptors may be caused not only by the rise in temperature but also by the increase in ionic strength to 0.4 M. The addition of ammonium sulfate,[4,5] molybdate ions[6] and a number of metals[7] to the incubation medium has an effect on the receptor activation process and accelerates the formation of the hormone-receptor complex.

It should be taken into consideration that the concentration of the steroid-receptor complex is also dependent on the equilibrium of the activation reaction of the receptor. In experiments *in vitro*, it was shown that there was a dynamic equilibrium between the number of activated and nonactivated receptor molecules. For cytoplasmic receptors (an ionic strength of 0.05 M KCl, pH 7.4, and a protein concentration of 8 mg/ml), the equilibrium in the reaction of activation comes at the ratio of 60% activated molecules and 40% nonactivated molecules. The equilibrium in the reaction of activation may be altered *in vitro* by many factors (pH, various salts, low molecular inhibitors); however their degree of influence *in vivo* is not clear.[8]

Such a variety of influences, which lead to a conformational change in the receptor structure, make it possible to form a hypothesis on the presence of a low molecular inhibitor (which is bound to the receptor and prevents its conversion to an active form). The search for such an inhibitor led to the isolation of a heat-resistant substance which could prevent the receptor transition to the active form. From the evidence, pyridoxal phosphate has surfaced as a potential inhibitor.[8] Some works recently published show that molybdate can inhibit receptor activation as well.[6,9]

Hence, many factors have shown that the mechanism of receptor activation is associated with a reversible reconstruction of their molecular structure. This leads to the ability of the activated molecules to migrate to a nucleus and, with an increased affinity, a contact center for acceptor sites localized in intranuclear structures.

By examining the process of cytoplasmic androgen receptor activation, the interaction of a hormone with a receptor should be considered to be a primary stimulus initiating this process. It is this contact of hormone with receptor molecule acceptor center that can cause the separation of a low molecular inhibitor, a structural reconstruction of receptor molecule, and the opening of the center allowing interaction with chromatin structures. Therefore, the presence of a hormone serves as a factor determining the transition of free, nonactivated androgen receptor forms to "occupied" activated hormone-receptor complexes. It should also be noted that there exist some data that show the possibility of a receptor molecule activation in the absence of the hormone.[10]

The activation process stipulated by its intramolecular reconstruction, and the opening of the center which is able to interact with chromatin structures, might be reversible. The functional significance of the receptor activation is associated first with the process of hormone-receptor complex migration from cytoplasm to cellular nucleus (although the mechanism of such a translocation is not clear) and, second, developing the properties which are necessary for binding this complex to chromatin. As the observations demonstrate in the process of receptor activation, the location of ionic charged groups on its surface changes. It leads to a redistribution of the charges, thereby increasing the possibility of interaction with various polyanions forming a part of chromatin.

The receptors of steroid hormones represent a group of proteins having the ability for a high degree of modification by means of phosphorylation, methylation and acetylation of separate functional groups. Quite a number of attempts have been made to elucidate the functional necessity of such a high modification of hormone-steroid receptors. Perhaps the most successful investigations were those which revealed the bond between the ATP level in cells and the ability of the receptor to form complexes with steroids.[11,12] The dependence of the strength of steroid binding by cytoplasmic receptors on the state of energy-dependent processes in the cell and the level of ATP showed the possibilities of receptor phosphorylation. In recent years, investigators have shown that cytoplasmic receptors of a number of steroid hormones may be attributed to phosphoproteins.[13,14] The data showed that in the presence of sodium molybdate, or sodium fluorite, it was possible to attain higher values of steroid-hormone binding. This served as a precondition for developing the investigations on cytoplasmic receptor phosphorylation. To completely confirm these preconditions, the isolation of phosphorylated forms of cytoplasmic receptors is needed. The purification of progesterone receptors of hen oviducts on DEAE-Sepharose resulted in two fractions of receptors with a sedimentation constant of 8 S. During electrophoresis in PAAG with DS-Na it was shown that the first fraction had a molecular mass of 90,900 and it included the ^{32}P-labile component. Two proteins were revealed in the structure of the second fraction: one protein with the same molecular mass (90,000 daltons) and another with a molecular mass of 10,400 daltons. In each of these proteins ^{32}P turned out to be bound to serins.[14] Direct evidence of phosphorylation of glucocorticoid receptors was obtained in experiments on L-cells from which two fractions of phosphorylated receptors with a molecular mass of 92,000 and 100,000 daltons were also isolated.[15–17]

Numerous investigations have shown that in cytoplasm, under the action of the enzyme Ca^{2+} and calmodulin-dependent protein kinase in the presence of ATP, there occurs the phosphorylation of a receptor which turns into an activated state and forms a hormone-receptor complex.[13,18] Perhaps the most convincing evidence of the possibility of steroid hormone receptor phosphorylation was obtained in experiments with purified glucocorticoid receptors. It was shown that by incubating a receptor (with a molecular weight of 90,000) in the presence of $\gamma\,^{32}$P-ATP and Mo^{2+}, phosphorylation of the protein occurs without adding exogenous enzyme of protein kinase.[19] In this way, for the first time, it was shown that glucocorticoid receptors possess phosphoprotein kinase activity and in the presence of a hormone (dexamethasone) and ATP, it was possible to carry out the phosphorylation of its several functional groups. The phosphorylation of a receptor molecule leads to its modification and allowed for the possibility of a transition to the activated state with the formation of a hormone-receptor complex. The comparison of some kinetic characteristics of phosphoprotein kinase activity of glucocorticoid receptors with specific nuclear protein kinases shows their similarity. Thus, the discovery of phosphoprotein kinase activity in the molecular structure revealed the tight association between the receptor activation process and the formation of a hormone-receptor complex possessing intracellular energetic metabolism.

One can also note that the study of the processes of the phosphorylation of steroid hormone receptors revealed the participation of a few amino acids (not only serine and threonine,[13,20] but also tyrosine).[21,22] The tyrosine phosphorylation in the structure of protein molecules is becoming one of the important reactions of protein modification participating in cellular metabolic regulation. In addition to enzymes taking part in the processes of receptor phosphorylation, the possibility of the dephosphorylation of steroid hormone receptors was demonstrated. It was established that the incubation of cytosol fractions reduced the ability of receptors to bind glucocorticoids.[23] Our experiments with cytoplasmic androgen receptors isolated from rat skeletal muscles also established the reduction of binding ability of 19-nortestosterone and ^{3}H-testosterone during receptor incubation with highly purified nuclear phosphoprotein phosphatase. The effect of enzymes on steroid binding activity of androgen receptors is dependent on pH and is not conditioned by their temperature inactivation. The influence of phosphoprotein phosphatase is removed by means of preliminary enzyme heating for 15 min at 85°C and the addition of inhibitors NaF and Na_2MoO_4 (unpublished data). These data confirm the participation of androgen receptor phosphorylation processes in keeping a high level of hormones bound. Similar results were obtained on estradiol receptors which considerably decreased the binding activity under the influence of nuclear phosphatase[24] and reduced it in the presence of ATP-dependent protein kinase.[25] Hence, these findings testified to the presence of steroid hormone receptors of phosphatase groups which actively participate in the process of interaction with the hormone. Receptors dephosphorylated by phosphatases considerably decreases their ability for steroid binding.

The question of the functional significance of phosphorylated groups in receptor molecule modification has yet to be solved. A suggested hypothesis involves the process of receptor phosphorylation and its tight association with energetic metabolism in cytoplasm, leading to the formation of an activated receptor form, thus allowing the binding of the hormone and migration to the nuclei. The participation of phosphorylation and dephosphorylation processes in the modification of receptor functions will be examined in more detail by discussing receptor cycle.

The most complete information on the processes of cytoplasmic androgen receptor migration to cellular nuclei was obtained by studying basic androgen-dependent tissues (primarily ventral prostate). No outstanding evidence has yet been obtained for the existence of a nuclear androgen receptor in skeletal muscles. This is mainly due to certain technical difficulties which appear during the investigation of metabolism in this tissue. The need to discover the mechanism of AAS action at a molecular level necessitated the improvement of methods in order to study the peculiarities of AAS metabolism in the separate subcellular structure of skeletal muscles. An investigation of the principal stages of AAS action in skeletal muscles was carried out in our laboratory. The behavior of androgen receptors for a whole period of separate AAS action was observed. It was noted in Chapter 3 that the cytoplasmic androgen receptors allowed the formation of specific hormone-receptor complexes with AAS in skeletal muscles. From this the number of possible binding sites could be determined. The findings show that the content of androgen receptor binding sites which can be occupied by AAS in skeletal muscle cytoplasm is less than that in other androgen-dependent tissues. To elucidate the possibilities of hormone-receptor complex migration from cytoplasm to nucleus, we carried out some experiments involving ^{3}H-19-nortestosterone binding by skeletal muscle nuclei. The analysis of ^{3}H-19-nortestosterone binding by skeletal muscle nuclei carried out according to the Scatchard method showed that the points were disposed linearly and attested to the homogeneity of binding sites, in the presence of the receptors, to interact with hormones. This was confirmed by the determination of the value K_d which made up 11.2 ± 2.5 nM. The number of nuclear receptor binding sites made up 24.1 ± 1.7 fmol/mg of DNA.

To reveal the stereospecificity of nuclear androgen receptors toward separate steroid hormones, the binding of ^{3}H-19-nortestosterone by isolated nuclei in the presence of different concentrations of unlabeled steroids was investigated.

It was established that only AAS and androgens effectively suppressed ^{3}H-19-nortestosterone binding (Figure 11). Estradiol and progesterone may be attributed to weak competitors. Glucocorticoids have practically no interaction with nuclear androgen receptors. The calculation of the values of the relative competitive ability allowed the arrangement of the investigated steroids into the

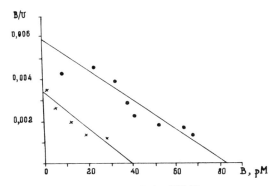

FIGURE 10. Scatchard analysis of ^{3}H-19-nortestosterone binding by androgen receptors in rat skeletal muscle nuclei and with 0.4 M KCl extract of nuclei ($\times$)

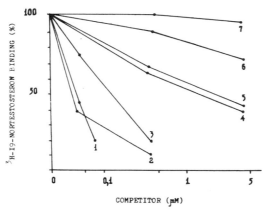

FIGURE 11. Competition of various steroids for ^{3}H-19-nortestosterone specific binding to the rat skeletal muscle nuclear androgen receptor. 19-Nortestosterone, 1; 5α-dihydrotestosterone, 2; testosterone, 3, progesterone, 4; 17β-estradiol, 5; dexamethasone, 6; corticosterone, 7.

following order: 5α-dihydrotestosterone > 19-nortestosterone > testosterone > estradiol > progesterone > dexamethasone > corticosterone.

The obtained characteristics of ligand specificity for nuclear and cytoplasmic androgen receptors in skeletal muscle practically coincide. This fact may be considered to be one of the essential pieces of evidence of the genesis of the nuclear form of androgen receptors from cytoplasmic forms in skeletal muscle as well as for other androgen-dependent tissues.[26,27]

After cytoplasmic androgen receptor activation and formation of the hormone-receptor complex, the process of migration to the nucleus occurs. It is accompanied by essential molecule reconstruction that is a receptor transformation. By comparing principal physical-chemical properties of androgen receptors, isolated from cytoplasm and prostate nuclei, it was established that in the process of the transformation, the receptor molecular mass changed. This was indicated by a reduction in the sedimentation coefficient during the centrifugation of the gradient of saccharose density. As was noted,[26] the cytoplasmic androgen receptor sedimentation constant was 3.8 S, while for the nuclear receptor it was 3.0 S, the isoelectric point of these receptors simultaneously changing.

As shown in Table 8, androgen receptors were revealed in various androgen-dependent organs. In the cytosol of these tissues there are receptors with a sedimentation coefficient of 8 to 9 S and a molecular mass of 200,000 to 300,000 daltons. When the ionic strength rises to 0.5 M KCl, they dissociate into 4 to 5 S form and the size of receptor molecules diminishes. There have been only a few preliminary studies that have looked at the nuclear form of androgen receptors. They have found a lower size of receptor molecule in comparison with cytoplasmic forms.

TABLE 8
Sizes of Androgen Receptors in Various Rat Tissues

Tissue	Receptor	Sedimentation coefficient	Radius of stokes (nm)	Molecular weight (daltons)	Ref.
Prostate	Cytoplasmic	8.0	8.4	276,000	28
		4.4	4.8	86,000	30
Liver		4.0	6.1	102,000	29
Prostate	Nuclear	2.9	2.2	26,500	27
Epididymis		3.0	2.2	26,000	27
Seminal vesicles		3.3	2.0	35,000	27

Great variation can be seen in the size of androgen receptor molecular weight and is associated with a different degree of proteolytic activity in various tissues. Proteases from rat prostate actively participating in androgen receptor splitting may be suppressed by specific inhibitors of serine-thiol protease.[33] As the findings indicate, the addition of molybdate stabilizes the androgen-receptor complex in an aggregated, untransformed state and protects it from dissociation. At the same time, molybdate acts as an inhibitor of the receptor transformation caused by the rise of salt concentration in the incubating solution.[9,34]

The translocation of the androgen-receptor complexes to nuclei leads to their interaction with different nuclear structures and to a gradual saturation of nuclear binding sites. The velocity of androgen-receptor complex accumulation in the nucleus is proportional to the concentration of such complexes in cytoplasm. The binding of the hormone-receptor complex in nuclei is characterized by a high affinity and a limited number of binding sites that limit the number of receptors in the nucleus. The transport of androgen receptor complexes to nuclei and their interaction with structural components inside nuclei have been most clearly demonstrated in prostate as a basic androgen-dependent organ. Experiments with isolated prostate nuclei have shown that they contain a limited number of sites of androgen binding. Using the extraction with salt solution of 0.05 to 0.1 *M* KCl, it made up 2000 to 3000 per nuclei cell with respect to one binding site for one receptor for one hormone molecule. According to a prostate functional state, the number of androgen receptor binding sites changes, and in the nuclei of hyperplasmic glands, it increases to 10,000, while after castration it decreases to 1000.

Extracted from ventral prostate nuclei, epididymis and seminal vesicles in salt solution, androgen receptors are similar in size to cytoplasmic receptors, isolated in salt solutions with a high ionic strength.[27] The purification of such receptors by means of gel chromatography with subsequent column chromatography on phosphocellulose showed three forms of receptors which differ in ion-exchangeable groups and molecular sizes. Androgen receptors are characterized by the dipole distribution of their electric charge. They belong to acidic proteins with an isoelectric point of 5.8. Androgen receptors, separated by means of column chromatography, are bound to anion-exchange resins containing diethylaminoethyl or other positively charged groups and are eluted with different salt concentrations in a polydispersed form. At neutral pH, androgen receptors are also bound to cation-exchange groups containing phosphate, carboxylmethyl, and glycine groups. Such a dipole behavior is typical for less than 1% of cytoplasmic proteins and these peculiarities may be of essential significance for an interaction process with nuclear structural components.

For androgen receptor purification, not only the basic methods of protein chemistry, but also some new biospecific methods are used. They are developed according to some peculiarities of receptor properties. The preferred method is a semiaffine purification method which uses either DNA-cellulose or DNA-Sepharose as a sorbent. However, as the evidence shows, the most promising method of androgen receptor isolation may be affinity chromatography on a matrix with a fixed steroid. The successive use of two synthetic affine sorbents of DNA-Sepharose 4B and testosterone-hemisuccinate-3,3-diamine propylamine-Sepharose 4B allowed the purification of the androgen receptor from seminal vesicles 540,000 times that of other methods.[35] This method of purification of an androgen receptor appeared to be rather effective, purifying 3 mg of pure protein from bull seminal vesicles. Investigating its physical-chemical properties, it was shown that according to a stereospecificity of binding to androgen receptor, the hormones are set in the following order: methyltrienolone > testosterone > 5α-dihydrotestosterone > 3β-hydroxy-Δ^5-androstan-17-one. K_d for methyltrienolone is 1.3 nM and for testosterone and is 4.0 nM.[35]

The first investigations on the purification of steroid hormone receptors having been carried out, the possibility of their practical use as antigens for obtaining specific antisera became evident. To accomplish this task we investigated the possibility of obtaining polyclonal antisera for steroid hormone receptors.[36–40] The presence of antisera considerably improved the methods of investigating hormone receptors. Some new methods in the study of receptor structure and their functions, irrespective of their ability for binding a radioactive ligand, were found. However the analysis of receptor molecule structure is limited by the heterogeneity and a low titer of polyclonic antisera. Another result from this new method of investigation was obtaining monoclonal antibodies for progesterone and estradiol receptors.[41,42] The use of the technology with hybridomes helped to isolate large quantities of monospecific immunoglobulins which are more effective than polyclonal antibodies isolated from animal serum. One of the first successes in using monoclonal antibodies was the discovery of the capability of a hormone-receptor-antibody complex to penetrate a nucleus. It was established that the translocation process of a hormone-receptor complex bound to monospecific immunoglobulin proceeds without any considerable alteration.[41] While studying the structure and the mechanism of steroid hormone receptor action, from the perspective of using monoclonal antibodies, one can see the possibilities of this scientific trend.

After migration to a cellular nucleus, the androgen-receptor complex interacts with various structural components localized in it. Among intranuclear structures such as nuclear membrane of karyoplasm, nuclear matrix, nucleole, and chromatin, the hormone-receptor complex is most tightly bound to chromatin. At the same time, some of these complexes may be localized in nuclear matrix or karyoplasm. Their presence might be stipulated by the dissociation of hormone-receptor complexes with chromatin. In most cases, the findings show that chromatin is the basic place of localization of hormone-receptor complexes in the nucleus. Experiments on cell free systems have revealed DNA interaction with hormone-receptor complexes. The ability of DNA to bind androgen-receptor complexes is shown in different ways.[43,46]

In recent years, there has been a certain amount of success in the study of chromatin structure and function in nuclear cells of eukaryotes.[40,41,47,50] Besides DNA, chromatin has five fractions of histones (H2A, H2B, H3, H4 and H1), some hundreds of nonhistone proteins, RNA, and lipids that form complexes. The ratio of histones and DNA (1:1) in chromatin of various tissues is relatively constant while the ratio of DNA and nonhistone proteins, as well as DNA and RNA, varies within large limits. The principal role of histones is associated with chromatin and its structural organization into nucleosomes and supernucleosomal structures. The nonhistone proteins not only participate in forming a chromatin structure, but they also act as a regulator function, ensuring a number of enzyme reactions in the nucleus and a specificity of an interaction of chromatin components. In the chromatin structure there is RNA which makes up 10 to 12% of the DNA content and varies considerably according to molecular weight. Parallel with a new synthesized pre-mRNA and pre-pRNA in the chromatin structure, there are low molecular weight RNAs; however, their functional role has not been clearly established. Lipids in chromatin make up only 1 to 2%, and they are represented mainly by sphingomyelin, phosphatidylcholine and phosphatidylethanolamine. The main part of chromatin is made up of DNA, its quantity being the constant value for all the cells of this kind of organism.

Three levels of DNA organization have been established: nucleosomal, chromomere and chromosomal.[51] The first level of DNA organization is associated with chromatin, which consists of separate subunits known as nucleosomes. An octamer histone complex is formed by four pairs of H2A, H2B, H3 and H4 molecules; one molecule of H1 histone and a DNA fragment of about 145 ± 7 base pairs form a part of the nucleosome. The core, which is universal for all the nucleosomes, consists of a histone octamer and a DNA fragment forming 1.75 turns of a left superhelix on the surface of the nucleosome. The nucleosome, a type of a filament 10 nm thick, represents the first level of chromatin organization. At the next level of organization the nucleosome filament curls up into a fibril 25 nm thick. Finally, this fibril forms a chain of loops which appears to be a structural-functional unit of chromatin domain.[49] At present there is a certain amount of evidence concerning the location of histones along the DNA chain, as well as the formation of pins which include turned nucleotide sequences known as palindromes.

Chromatin DNA is heterogeneous according to its structure and is represented by three kinds of nucleotide sequences: unique (nonrepeated), moderately repetitive, and frequently repetitive. The unique sequences of DNA nucleotides pertain to structural genes and include information on structural and functional proteins. They are transcribed as heterogeneous nuclear RNA (hnRNA) in which all pre-mRNA form their parts. Moderately repetitive sequences of DNA nucleotides represent regulator genome centers from which the transcription of regulator RNA participating in the conversion of pre-mRNA occurs. A considerable part of often repetitive sequences of DNA nucleotides is transcribed in the structure of hnRNA. Their role consists of interaction with specific molecules (protein and DNA) which regulate the activity of structural genes adjoining them. A great number of pin structures in DNA and their derivatives, as well as their ability for transcription, demonstrate their great functional significance in eukaryote genomes. The chromatin sites which are at the stage of active transcription have some peculiarities of structure in comparison with non-transcribed chromatin. The active chromatin is characterized by a lesser compactness, a high sensitivity to the action of endogenous enzymes and often by an alteration of chromatin structure.

Gene transcription begins with the recognition of promotor centers by RNA polymerase which then moves along the DNA molecule, synthesizing the RNA molecule with the sequence of complementary gene sequence until the enzyme reaches the terminator sequence (Figure 12).

The velocity of the formation and the quantity of various proteins which are necessary for accomplishing a specific function in the cell may be regulated at several stages. First is the transcription of pre-mRNA on chromatin. Second is a processing of pre-mRNA conversion to mRNA that allows transcription to occur. Third, there is a mRNA translation in the ribosome. Finally, there is a process of limited proteolysis of synthesized proteins. One of the main stages of the regulation process in the transmission of genetic information is carried out at the level of transcription. The size of a complete gene is larger than the value of the mRNA coding of a definite protein. Inside the gene there are one or more nucleotide sequences of different length which were called introns. They pass

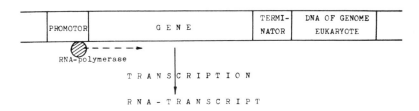

FIGURE 12. General diagram of transcribed gene.

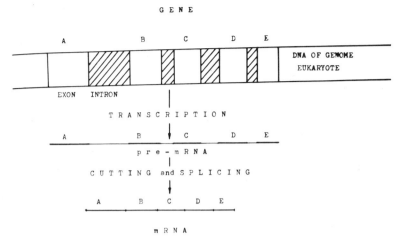

FIGURE 13.   Diagram of gene eukaryote organizing and RNA transcript processing.

information only to the pre-mRNA. These are the sequences which code the RNA fragments that are being removed in the process of mRNA maturation. The mRNA receives information only from DNA nucleotide sequences which are called exons. The molecules of pre-mRNA are precursors of real mRNA where, in the nucleus, they are subjected to a limited hydrolysis and splicing. As a result, nucleotide sequences corresponding to introns are cut out and exon sequences are sewn together (Figure 13).

To reveal the mechanism of hormone-receptor complex action at the level of gene expression, molecular-biological investigations in several principal directions have been carried out in recent years. The investigations on the receptor interaction with specific DNA nucleotide sequences are of considerable importance. For this reason one uses the cloning of separate genes with the help of plasmids, as well as the phenomenon of transfection. Thus one can use nucleic acids of separate viruses, in particular the mouse mammary tumor virus (MMTV).[52,53] The merits of such a model are evident. It allows the study of a number of specific DNA fragments, which exist around structural genes, and shows the possibility of binding the hormone-receptor complex to it after translocation to the nucleus. The other trend includes the study of the process of transcription *in vitro* on reconstructed systems in the presence of the hormone-receptor complex.[54]

By studying the distribution of acceptor activity in separate chromatin fractions, after extraction with salt solutions of diverse concentration, it is shown that androgen-receptor complexes may interact with three fractions of nonhistone proteins.[55] The role of nonhistone proteins as factors determining the ability of chromatin to interact with androgen receptors is distinctly revealed in the experiments on reconstructed homologous and heterologous chromatin using different fractions of nonhistone proteins. It was shown that the basic binding activity of nonhistone acid proteins is concentrated in the fraction extracted with 0.35 M KCl. These are the proteins that are associated with actively transcribed chromatin sequences. The participation of specific chromosomal proteins and DNA sequences in the interaction processes with androgen-receptor complexes in various tissues is reflected in detail in a very thorough review.[56] By fractionating the nonhistone proteins of chromatin, the main objective was to attempt to find an individual protein which determines the binding ability with androgen-receptor complex and has the necessary acceptor center. The successive purification in DNA-cellulose columns resulted in the isolation of protein which actively interacts with androgen receptor. During electrophoresis in PAAG, such an acceptor protein was seen to migrate in the form of a stripe (mw = 14,000 daltons). An analysis of the amino acid composition showed a predominance of acidic amino acid. The functional activity of this acceptor protein was tested on the reconstructed cell free system by including ATP and GTP in a newly synthesized RNA. The principal role of such an acceptor protein, which binds the androgen receptor, is to initiate pre-mRNA synthesis by gene expression.[35,36,57,58] These findings show that besides acidic and basic nonhistone proteins of chromatin, DNA can also participate directly in androgen-receptor complex binding.[59,60] The receptors binding to DNA proceed as an electrostatic interaction which decreases with increasing ionic strength.[61–63] The abundant evidence testifies to a nonspecific character of steroid-receptor binding to pure DNA. There was no evidence to show differences in steroid-receptor complex binding to native DNA from different kinds of animals.[64–66] The process of receptor interaction with pure DNA does not have a saturated character.[56,67] Nonspecific steroid receptors binding to DNA with a low affinity may essentially prevent revealing a small quantity of genome acceptor binding sites to which the transmission of a hormonal signal is directed.[68] Several approaches to find the most practical way to analyze the specific acceptor sites of genome for steroid hormones have been offered. Experiments with progesterone receptors in cells infected with a tumor virus of mouse mammary gland are considered to be one of the most plausible methods. It turns out that under these conditions, progesterone regulates the velocity of genome virus transcription. This fact led to some very refined and promising experiments which resulted in the cloning of virose DNA and the determination of the fragments of such DNA which specifically binds a progesterone-receptor complex. The use of adsorption methods of complexes (hormone-receptor-fragment-DNA) on nitrocellulose filters showed that a highly purified progesterone receptor selectively interacted with the fragments of cloned DNA.[69] This approach made it possible to demonstrate at least one DNA fragment where there is a specific acceptor center binding the hormone-receptor complex, which is situated close to the starting point of RNA synthesis.[52] For direct interaction of a receptor with DNA, the presence of 250 to 300 pairs of nucleotides is needed.[44] From this sphere of nucleotidal DNA sequences, the acceptor center containing only 19 nucleotides, which specifically bound the receptor of progesterone,[70] was successfully isolated. However, the number of such acceptor sites on a genome proved to be rather limited, which made it difficult to explain their functional meaning.[60] The discovery of specific acceptor centers for steroid hormones in the structure of separate genes is undoubtedly of great importance for elucidating the mechanism of modulation and the expression of the genes which are under the control of steroid hormones. The most striking example of such investigations is the apparent finding of two centers in the terminal region of the DNA, the promoter binding the steroid-receptor complex, one of which is between 202 to 137 pairs of nucleotides while the other is between 137 to 50 pairs of nucleotides.[60] The presence of such specific sites on the DNA molecule for hormone-receptor complex in the promoter region allows the transmission of the hormone signal to regulate gene activity separately. One of the hypotheses explaining the mechanism of recognizing specific binding sites by receptors on chromatin is considered to be the possibility of a participating inhibitor protein closing the acceptor site.[54]

The process of androgen-receptor complex interaction with chromatin acceptor sites assumes not only the reaction of component association, but also the reaction of dissociation when the hormone-receptor complex is released from chromatin. The study of the kinetics of these reactions has shown that the reaction of association proceeded intensively enough, and the process of hormone-receptor binding to chromatin occurred within 10 min.[71] The release of this complex from chromatin, that is the reaction of dissociation, proceeds much more slowly — up to 70 minutes. During this period of time, the hormone-receptor complex actively participates in genome expression and just such a long binding to chromatin is important to allow enough time for a hormonal response.

After its completion the hormone-receptor complex is released from chromatin. As one of the potential mechanisms of a hormone-receptor complex being released from chromatin, it is hypothesized that nuclear RNA is bound to the receptor complex and facilitates its dissociation from chromatin acceptor sites. Conversely, the hormone-receptor complex itself is able to actively participate in RNA processing (stabilization and utilization). Experimental proof of such a hypothesis was obtained by androgen-receptor complexes binding to ribonucleoproteids or RNA may effectively release enough androgen-receptor complexes from DNA or nuclei. The ability of RNA to interact with a receptor complex depends on the nucleotide sequence and the polymeride size. The possibility of an androgen-receptor complex binding to RNA is shown not only in prostate, but also in mouse kidneys.

Evidence for a mechanism of hormone-receptor complex dissociation with subsequent receptor inactivation and hormonal release is still incomplete. However this process is reversible and dependent on the state of energetic reactions in the nucleus. The reduction of androgen-binding activity in the receptor proceeds very fast, without any loss in the total number of receptors and with an active ATP participating. The androgen molecules protect the receptor against inactivation. The nuclear androgen-receptor complex is inactivated much more slowly than the cytoplasmic hormone-receptor complex.[68] After the hormone-receptor complex dissociates, a fraction of free nonactivated receptors is formed in the nucleus and is in a dynamic equilibrium with a fraction of the free cytoplasmic receptors. The process of dephosphorylation may be important in the mechanism of receptor inactivation. This reaction occurs with the participation of nuclear phosphoprotein phosphatase and can considerably change the receptor binding properties. It was shown that during saturation with 17β-estradiol, the estrogen nuclear receptor is inactivated by phosphoprotein phosphatase.[74] However, if instead of the hormone the receptor is saturated with antihormones of a nonsteroid nature (nafoxidie or tamoxifen), then the enzyme does not interact with such a complex and the period of its life is longer than that of the receptor with the estradiol complex. The presence of phosphoprotein phosphatase in the nuclei of liver and kidney cells, as well as in the nuclei of androgen-dependent tissues and in the epithelium of seminal vesicles, confirms the possibility of its participation in the processes of receptor dephosphorylation.[75]

The fate of these free nuclear receptors can take two pathways:

1. Their direct return from the nucleus to the cytoplasm, or
2. A repeated receptor reactivation in the nucleus which occurs with the participation of energy-dependent processes with repeated hormone binding and an interaction with chromatin.

Such intranuclear androgen receptor conversions have been confirmed experimentally.[71]

The possible role of the nucleus structural components in the mechanism of interaction with an androgen-receptor complex has led to the participation of not only chromatin, but also other nuclear structures in this process. The calculations show that for the saturation of the nucleus binding capacity, which is determined in 10^4 receptors, the participation of numerous nuclear structures is needed. Such a binding of hormone-receptor complexes in the nucleus is characterized by a low affinity and may considered to be nonspecific to a large extent. It has been demonstrated in experiments on nuclei *in vivo*,[64] *in vitro*,[65] as well as on DNA.[66]

Specific androgen-binding sites have been shown to exist in nuclear membranes[76] and nuclear matrices.[77] The nuclear matrix contains two structures: a nuclear envelope, or fibrous layer (lamina), bound to porous complexes and an intranuclear fibrillar or granular net. Within the structure of the nuclear matrix, proteins prevail (96%); however, there are also phospholipids (1.5 to 2%) and some trace amounts of DNA and RNA. The proteins in the nuclear matrix consist of nonhistone proteins with a high level of turnover, and in the phospholipids a fraction of sphingomyelin prevails. The nuclear matrix plays not only a structural role in the cellular nucleus skeleton, but it also actively participates in DNA initiation and replication, synthesis, RNA processing and transport, and hormone-receptor complex binding including androgen receptors.[78] In the nuclei of the ventral prostate, the nuclear matrix contains approximately half of the androgen-binding sites.[79] Improvements in the technique of analyzing androgen receptor binding ability results in higher values of nuclei androgen-binding capacity. Ignoring the methods of salt extraction, the use of nuclei processing by means of ultrasound and proteolytic and nuclease enzymes considerably increases the number of androgen binding sites in nuclei. As a result, the number of androgen binding sites in the nuclei from ventral prostate may be from 18,000 to 23,000 molecules. That is an extraction 10 to 20 times greater than with only a salt solution of 0.05 to 0.1 M KCl.[80,81] This pertains to androgen receptors with a sedimentation constant of 3 S, which are bound tightly enough to the nuclear matrix that they can only be seen after the nuclei have been processed by nucleases and trypsin. The differences between androgen receptor extraction are stipulated not only by their location in various nuclear structures, but also by how long the bonds last. Thus, we can distinguish two intranuclear receptors, approximately equal by their quantity fractions. The first group of androgen receptors contains 10,000 molecules. After a light digestion with micrococcal nuclease and extraction with 0.6 M NaCl, it may be removed out of intranuclear structures (mainly chromatin). The second group of receptors is more strongly bound to the nuclear matrix. It contains 8000 to 13,000 molecules and is released only after digestion with trypsin.[81]

The ability of nuclei to bind androgen-receptor complexes in other tissues, which have a low sensitivity to androgen action, is considerably less. The results of determining androgens and AAS nuclear binding in skeletal muscles may be considered to be the proof of this thesis (Table 9). One can see that skeletal muscle nuclei have the ability to bind androgens; however, to date there has been no experimental evidence to support this view and some skepticism has been expressed about the possibility of identifying androgen nuclear binding in skeletal tissues.

While studying the mechanism of AAS receptor binding in skeletal muscles, it was considered whether there exists the possibility of such a hormone-receptor complex transport to nuclei and their interaction with intracellular structures.

The following series of experiments shows that according to extraction with salt solutions of various concentrations, nuclear androgen receptors from rat

TABLE 9

The Concentration of Nuclear Androgen Receptor Binding Sites in Skeletal Muscles

Nuclei components	K_d(nM)	B_{max} (fmol/mg DNA)	Ref.
Intact nuclei	6–8	151	79
	11.2	24	83
0.4 M KCl extract	9.9	55	83
Nuclear matrix	2–3	56	82

skeletal muscles may be divided into three fractions. The first, easily released, fraction of receptors is isolated by the concentration of 0.25 M KCl and it probably represents the receptors which are mainly free from hormones. The second receptor fraction is extracted from the nuclei with a solution of 0.4 M KCl and represents slowly dissociating hormone-receptor complexes extracted from chromatin.

The third fraction of androgen receptors dissolves with a solution of 1.0 M KCl during extraction. If the first two androgen receptor fractions, according to their localization, may be attributed with certainty to receptor complexes interacting with chromatin, then the receptors which are insoluble during salt extraction might be bound to the nuclear matrix.

In spite of considerable difficulties that are inevitably caused from the interpretation of the data obtained in the experiments with nuclear androgen receptors, these findings nevertheless indicate that

1. Androgen receptors may be in a free or bound to a hormone state in the nucleus, and
2. Receptor molecules have functional groups or centers which allow binding to DNA, RNA, nonhistone proteins of chromatin, and nuclear matrix.

The functional necessity of such a heterogeneous receptor location in the nucleus has not been clearly established and needs special study.

By analyzing the mechanism of AAS nuclear binding in skeletal muscle, one should take into consideration that androgen-selective nuclear binding has also been shown to exist in marrow.[84] It has been demonstrated that after extraction of 0.5 M KCl, the androgen binding protein, with a rather pronounced steroid specificity, was isolated from the purified nuclei of marrow.[85] The androgen receptor system in marrow cells includes only a specific binding of hormones in the nuclei and it does not reveal the presence of cytoplasmic receptors. These findings on androgen binding in marrow essentially differ from those obtained in other tissues. Additionally, they show the possibility of a specific androgen binding directly to a nucleus, which was also shown on the nuclei of skeletal muscles.[83] Thus, the possibility of a direct androgen interaction with a receptor solely in the nucleus appears to be rather convincing.

The comparison of separate stages of AAS interaction with androgen receptors in diverse intracellular structures formulates the notion of a receptor cycle. The idea of a closed receptor cycle has been raised in other investigations.[86,87] According to these investigations androgen receptor proteins make cyclic migrations between cytoplasm and nucleus. The hormone-receptor complex is translocated from the cytoplasm to the nucleus and then, after release from chromatin acceptor sites, the receptor together with the nuclear ribonucleoproteids is returned to cytoplasm and beings a new cycle. This hypothetical concept proved to be verisimilar enough and in the last 10 years it has received increasing support. Numerous investigations carried out on various tissues have shown that

1 to 4 hours after a hormone-receptor injection into an animal, the initial number of receptors in cytoplasm has been reduced.[88,89] The time of one receptor cycle varies considerably in different tissues and seems to depend on the hormone type, the method of injection, the dose, and the rate of metabolism for the given animal. The most widespread methodical approach in the analysis of a receptor cycle is the study of the receptor distribution after a single hormone injection. To estimate the receptor cycle in skeletal muscles, by saturating an organism with AAS we investigated temporal alterations of cytoplasmic and nuclear 19-nortestosterone binding after injecting a physiological dose of hormone. The results of the 19-nortestosterone binding in cytoplasm and skeletal muscle nuclei, as well as its content in rats' blood, are given in Figure 14.

After a hormone injection, the number of free cytoplasmic receptors rapidly reduces to 15 to 20% of the initial level. Such a decrease in the number of receptors is associated with their interaction with 19-nortestosterone and the translocation of hormone-receptor complexes to the nucleus. In 2 hours, an increase in receptor binding is observed and in 4 hours it twice exceeds the initial level. Such an increase in the number of cytoplasmic receptors is probably due to their return to cytoplasm. The maximum value of 19-nortestosterone nuclear binding was observed 2 hours after injection of the hormone. The change of 19-nortestosterone concentration in the blood has an impulsive character, with a maximum of 30 min after an injection. Four hours later the hormone concentra-

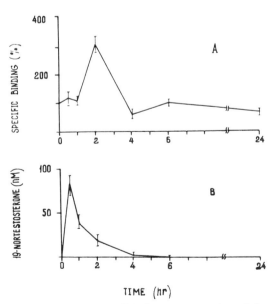

FIGURE 14.   Binding of ^{3}H-19-nortestosterone in rat skeletal muscle nuclei (A) and its concentration in blood (B) after hormone injection.

tion in the blood is practically reduced to zero. The findings obtained show that after a single injection of AAS-19-nortestosterone into the organism in skeletal muscles, there occurs a hormone binding to a receptor, the translocation of hormone-receptor complex to the nuclei, and the subsequent return to cytoplasm. The receptor cycle is completed 4 to 6 hours before free receptors migrate to the cytoplasm. It also should be noted that in this series of investigations we determined only the fractions of free androgen receptors. To have more precise characteristics of the receptor cycle it is necessary to know the total quantity of androgens (both free and occupied by a hormone).

Summing up the problems discussed in this chapter, it should be noted that we have accumulated a large quantity of experimental facts which demonstrate a scheme of biological processes ensuring the participation of receptors in the transmission of a hormonal signal into a cell.

The receptor cycle includes the following successive stages:

1. Transport of hormone to a cell.
2. Receptor activation, receptor phosphorylation, hormone-receptor complex formation.
3. Hormone-receptor complex translocation to the nucleus.
4. Hormone-receptor complex interaction with chromatin acceptor sites and hormone signal transmission.
5. Hormone-receptor complex release from chromatin, receptor dephosphorylation, dissociation to free receptor and hormone.
6. Transport of free receptor to cytoplasm, receptor splitting by cytoplasmic proteases.
7. Synthesis of new receptor molecules in cytoplasm.

The sequence of these possible events for the androgen receptor binding AAS in skeletal muscles is given in Figure 15.

One may note two peculiarities of this scheme which distinguish it from other similar investigations.[86,91] The first and very important peculiarity involves the association between the process of receptor activation accompanied by protein receptor phosphorylation and energetics of cell metabolism.[90,91]

At present a number of experimental corroborations of the binding of nucleoside triphosphates specific to receptor protein molecules have been obtained. This assumes the presence of specific ATP binding sites on the molecules of steroid hormone receptors. The possibility of a direct ATP interaction with intracellular receptor proteins for the receptors of progestins,[92] glucocorticoids,[93] estrogens[91] and androgens[45,94] has been shown. Direct experiments with ATP, immobilized on Sepharose, revealed binding sites of nucleotides in the molecules of steroid receptors. It turned out that ATP interacts with an inhibitor which is located within the structure of the receptor. As a resullt of molecule modification, the receptor turns into an activated state and its affinity for the hormone increases.[95] These results show that ATP can be considered as a specific

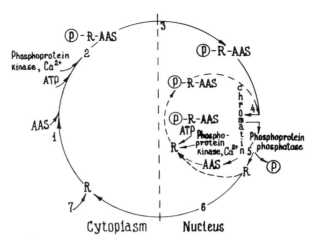

FIGURE 15.   Scheme of androgen receptors intracellular cycle in skeletal muscles. R, androgen receptor; P–R, activated receptor; P–R–AAS, hormone-receptor complex.

modulator of receptor activation and a regulator of the process of activated hormone-receptor complex translocation to the nuclei.[96,97]

The second peculiarity lies in the fact that the process of receptor inactivation is closely linked with the dephosphorylation of its molecule. After the release of hormone-receptor complex from chromatin under the action of the enzyme phosphoprotein phosphatase, a receptor dephosphorylation occurs which is then transported to cytoplasm.[18,91] One may hypothesize that a cyclic cascade of phosphorylation-dephosphorylation participates in nuclei receptor modification. The analysis of enzyme-reversible covalent modifications with the participation of such a cascade system demonstrates that it ensures extremely large regulated possibilities to enzymes.[98] In all probability, receptor proteins for steroid hormones in a cellular nucleus may also be subjected to a modification with the participation of the phosphorylation-dephosphorylation cyclic cascade system. The ability of such a cascade system to maintain the level of phosphorylated receptors depends on the supply of ATP providing the energy. The calculations show that under normal conditions, the cyclic cascade system consumes a very small quantity of energy in the form of ATP molecules and makes up less than 0.02% of the total energy expenditure in the nucleus.[99]

The use of monoclonal antibodies, as well as immunocytochemical methods, convincingly shows an exceptionally nuclear localization of estrogen receptors.[100–102] The high content of receptor proteins in cytoplasm, which has been revealed by biochemical methods, is bound up with a disturbance of nuclei structure by tissue homogenization. These results with regard to a two-stage pattern of hormonal signal transmission in a cell (the pattern which has become classical) come with a great deal of skepticism.[103,104] There has arisen a necessity of critical analysis of the extensive experimental evidence on the localization of steroid hormone receptors in the cell and on the role of various factors in the process of the formation and activation of hormone-receptor complexes.

The participation of protein kinases and phosphatases in the process of steroid hormone receptor phosphorylation and dephosphorylation as a necessary condition for the receptor to be in the activated state in the presence of hormone not only confirms the concept of a receptor cycle in the cell, but also turns it from an autonomous process to an energy-dependent process attended by a lot of reactions of accumulation and using an ATP cellular fund. Thus, the processes of hormonal and intercellular autonomic regulation are closely associated in a united biochemical mechanism of metabolic regulation in the organism.

Each of the stages of the receptor cycle distinguished in the scheme represents a complicated biochemical process which can be regulated by a number of factors. Today the participation of endogenetic regulators has been shown to occur in at least two stages. The first, a protein factor (the inhibitor of translation), interacts with hormone-receptor complex and oppresses its binding in the nuclei and in this way limits a specific hormone-binding capacity of the nuclei.[107,108] The study of the physical-chemical properties of this inhibitor revealed a few component polypeptides with a diverse molecular weight and various compositions of amino acids.[6,109] The process of androgen-receptor complex translocation may be blocked by introducing cyproterone acetate antiandrogens into the organism which selectively interact with the receptor.[110] The second protein factor accelerates the release of the androgen-receptor complex from chromatin acceptor sites.[111] Hence, the process of transmitting the hormonal signal to a cell at the stage of interaction with a receptor may be regulated not only by the relation of principal components (hormone and receptor), but also by a number of other factors tightly associated with intracellular metabolism.

The model of the receptor cycle does not exclude the possibility of the synthesis of a new receptor molecule which has found experimental confirmation in a number of works.[86,112] At the same time it shows the close association between androgen receptor functions, the regulation of their state in different intracellular structures (primarily in the nucleus with the principal reactions of energetic metabolism) and their close connection with the state of energy-dependent reactions, all of which are involved in a common integrated system of intracellular regulation.

REFERENCES

1. **Weichman, B. M. and Notides, A. C.,** Analysis of estrogen receptor activation by its (^{3}H)-estradiol dissociation kinetics, *Biochemistry,* 18, 220, 1979.
2. **Milgrom, E.,** Activation of steroid-receptor complexes, *Biochem. Actions Horm.,* 8, 465, 1981.
3. **Atgor, M. and Milgrom, E.,** Mechanism and kinetics of the thermal activation of glucocorticoid hormone receptor complex, *J. Biol. Chem.,* 251, 4758, 1976.

4. **Jensen, E. V., Mohla, S., and Garell, T.,** Estrophile to nucleophile in two easy steps, *J. Steroid Biochem.,* 3, 445, 1972.
5. **Giannopoulos, G.,** Glucocorticoid receptor in lung, *J. Biol. Chem.,* 250, 2904, 1975.
6. **Dahmer, M. K., Housley, P. R., and Pratt, W. B.,** Effects of molybdate and androgenous inhibitors on steroid-receptor inactivation, transformation and translocation, *Annu. Rev. Physiol.,* 46, 67, 1984.
7. **Hechter, O.,** The receptor concept: prejudice, prediction and paradox, in *Hormone Receptors,* Klacho, D.M. and Forte, L. R., Eds., Plenum Press, London, 1979.
8. **Bailley, A., Savouret, J. F., Sallas, N., and Milgrom, E.,** Factors modifying the equilibrium between activated and non-activated forms of steroid-receptor complexes, *Eur. J. Biochem.,* 88, 623, 1978.
9. **Nashigori, H. and Toft, D.,** Inhibition of progesterone receptor activation by sodium molybdate, *Biochemistry,* 19, 77, 1980.
10. **Buller, R. E., Toft, D. O., Schrader, W. T., and O'Malley, B. W.,** Progesterone-binding components of chick oviduct, *J. Biol. Chem.,* 250, 801, 1975.
11. **Munck, A. and Brinck-Johnsen, T.,** Specific and non-specific physicochemical interactions of glucocorticoids and related steroids with rat thymus cells in vivo, *J. Biol. Chem.,* 243, 5556, 1968.
12. **Sloman, J. C. and Bell, P. A.,** The dependence of specific nuclear binding of glucocorticoids by rat thymus cells on cellular ATP levels, *Biochim. Biophys. Acta,* 428, 403, 1976.
13. **Weigel, N. L., Tash, J. S., Means, A. R., Schradoe, W. T., and O'Malley, B. W.,** Phosphorylation of hen progesterone receptor by cAMP dependent protein kinase, *Biochem. Biophys. Res. Commun.,* 102, 513, 1981.
14. **Dougherty, J. J., Puri, P. K., and Toft, D. O.,** Phosphorylation in vivo of chicken oviduct progesterone receptor, *J. Biol. Chem.,* 257, 14226, 1982.
15. **Grandies, P., Miller, A., Schmidt, T., and Liftwack, G.,** Phosphorylation in vivo of rat hepatic glucocorticoid receptor, *Biochem. Biophys. Res. Commun.,* 120, 59, 1984.
16. **Sandro, J. J., Forest, A. C., and Pratt, W. B.,** ATP-dependent activation of L cell glucocorticoid receptors to the steroid binding form, *J. Biol. Chem.,* 254, 4772, 1979.
17. **Housley, P. R. and Pratt, W. B.,** Direct demonstration of glucocorticoid receptor phosphorylation by intact L-cells, *J. Biol. Chem.,* 258, 4630, 1983.
18. **Migliaccio, A., Lastorin, S., Moncharmont, R., Rotondi, A., and Auricchio, F.,** Phosphorylation of calf uterus 17β-estradiol receptor by endogenous Ca^{2+}-stimulated kinase activating the hormone binding of the receptor, *Biochem. Biophys. Res. Commun.,* 109, 1002, 1982.
19. **Kurl, R. N. and Jacob, S. T.,** Phosphorylation of purified glucocorticoid receptor from rat liver by an endogenous protein kinase, *Biochem. Biophys. Res. Commun.,* 119, 700, 1984.
20. **Leach, K. L., Dahmer, M. K., Hammond, N. D., Sando, J. J., and Pratt, W. B.,** Molybdate inhibition of glucocorticoid receptor inactivation and transformation, *J. Biol. Chem.,* 254, 11884, 1979.
21. **Gnosh-Dastidar, P. and Fox, C. F.,** Epidermal growth factor and epidermal growth factor receptor-dependent phosphorylation of a Mr-34000 protein substrate for pp 60[src], *J. Biol. Chem.,* 258, 2041, 1983.
22. **Gnosh-Dastidar, P., Coty, W. A., Griest, R. E., Wood, D. L., and Fox, C. F.,** Progesterone receptor subunits are high affinity substrates for phosphorylation by epidermal growth factor receptor, *Proc. Natl. Acad. Sci. USA,* 81, 1654, 1984.
23. **Nielson, C. J., Sando, J. J., and Pratt, W. B.,** Evidence that dephosphorylation inactivates glucocorticoid receptors, *Proc. Natl. Acad. Sci. USA,* 74, 1398, 1977.
24. **Auricchio, F., Migliaccio, A., and Rotondi, A.,** Inactivation of oestrogen receptor in vitro by nuclear dephosphorylation, *Biochem. J.,* 194, 569, 1981.
25. **Auricchio, F., Migliaccio, A., Castoria, S., Lastoria, S., and Rotondi, A.,** Evidence that in vivo oestradiol receptor translocated into nuclei is dephosphorylated and released into cytoplasm, *Biochem. Biophys. Res. Commun.,* 106, 149, 1982.

26. **Idao, S.,** Cellular receptors and mechanisms of action of steroid hormones, *Int. Rev. Cytol.,* 71, 87, 1975.

27. **Lea, O. A., Wilson, E. M., and French, F. S.,** Characterization of different forms of the androgen receptors, *Endocrinology,* 105, 1350, 1979.

28. **Mainwaring, W. I. P.,** A soluble androgen receptor in the cytoplasm of rat prostate, *J. Endocrinol.,* 45, 531, 1969.

29. **Gustasson, J.-Å., Pousette, A., and Stenberg, A.,** Intranuclear transport of androstandione in the rat liver, *J. Steroid Biochem.,* 8, 793, 1977.

30. **Bruchovsky, N., Rennie, P. S., Lessor, B., and Sutherland, J. A.,** The influence of androgen receptors on the concentration of androgens in nuclei of hormone-responsive cells, *J. Steroid Biochem.,* 6, 551, 1975.

31. **Hiipakka, R. A., Loor, R. M., and Idao, S.,** Receptors and factors regulating androgen action in the rat ventral prostate, in *Gene Regulation by Steroid Hormones,* Roy, A. K. and Clark, J. H., Eds., Springer-Verlag, New York, 1980. 194.

32. **Janne, O. A., Isoomaa, V. V., Piunen, A. E., Wright, W. W., and Bardin C. N.,** How changes in cytosol and nuclear androgen receptors relate to the testosterone responses: studies with new exchange assays, in *Gene Regulation by Steroid Hormones,* Roy, A. K. and Clark J. H., Eds., Springer-Verlag, New York, 1983, 277.

33. **Prins, G. S. and Lee, C.,** Effect of protease inhibitors on androgen receptor analysis in rat prostate cytosol, *Steroids,* 40, 3005, 1982.

34. **Rowley, D. R., Change, Ch. H., and Tindal, D. J.,** Effect of sodium molybdate on the androgen receptor from the P 3327 prostatic tumor, *Endocrinology,* 114, 1776, 1984.

35. **Change, C. H., Rowley, D. R., Lobl, T. J., and Tindal, D. J.,** Purification and characterization of androgen receptor from steer seminal vesicle, *Biochemistry,* 21, 4102, 1982.

36. **Greene, G. L., Fitsh, F. W., and Jensen, E. V.,** Monoclonal antibodies to estrophilin. Probes for the study of estrogen receptors, *Proc. Natl. Acad. Sci. USA,* 77, 5115, 1980.

37. **Greene, G. L., Nolan, C., Engler. J. P., and Jensen, E. V.,** Monoclonal antibodies to human estrogen receptor, *Proc. Natl. Acad. Sci. USA,* 7, 5115, 1980.

38. **Okret, S., Carldstedt-Duke, J., Wrange, O., Carlström, K., and Gustafsson, J.-O.,** Characterization of an antiserum against the glucocorticoid receptor, *Biochim. Biophys. Acta,* 677, 205, 1981.

39. **Carlstedt-Duke, J., Okret, S., Wrange, O., and Gustafsson, J.-O.,** Immunochemical analysis of the glucocorticoid receptor: identification of a third domain separate from the steroid-binding and DNA-binding domains, *Proc. Natl. Acad. Sci. USA,* 79, 4260, 1982.

40. **Okret, S.,** Comparison between different rabbit antisera against the glucocorticoid receptor, *J. Steroid Biochem.,* 19, 1241, 1983.

41. **Monchrmout, B., Su, J. L., and Parkh, I.,** Monoclonal antibodies against estrogen receptor: interaction with different molecular forms and functions of the receptor, *Biochemistry,* 21, 6916, 1982.

42. **Okret, S., Winstrom, A., Wrange, O., Andersson, B., and Gustafsson, J.-O.,** Monoclonal antibodies against the rat liver glucocorticoid receptor, *Proc. Natl. Acad. Sci. USA,* 81, 1609, 1984.

43. **Sluyser, M.,** Interaction of steroid hormone receptors with DNA, *Trends Biochem. Sci.,* 8, 236, 1983.

44. **Cato, A. C. B.,** How steroid hormones function to induce the transcription of specific genes, *Biosci. Rep.,* 3, 101, 1983.

45. **Mulder, E., Vrij, A. A., Brinkmann, A. O., Van der Molen, H. J., and Parker, M. C.,** Interaction of rat prostate androgen receptors with polynucleotides, RNA, DNA and cloned DNA fragments, *Biochim. Biophys. Acta,* 781, 121, 1984.

46. **Davies, P. and Thomas, P.,** Interaction of androgen receptors with chromatin and DNA, *J. Steroid Biochem.,* 20, 57, 1984.

47. **Gazarjan, K. G. and Tarantul, V. Z.,** *Eukaryotic Genome: Molecular Organization and Expression,* Moscow State University, Moscow, 1983.

48. **Kutscherenko, N. E., Tsudzevitch, B. A., Blum, Ja. B., and Babenjuk, Ju. D.,** *Biochemical Model of the Regulation of Chromatin Activity,* Naukova Dumka, Kiev, 1983.

49. **Igo-Kemenes, T., Hörz, W., and Lechon, H. G.,** Chromatin, *Annu. Rev. Biochem.,* 51, 89, 1982.

50. **Weisbrod, S.,** Active chromatin, *Nature,* 197, 280, 1982.

51. **Tarantul, V. Z., Goltsev, V. A., Kuznetsova, E. D.,** Structural organization of eukaryotic genome, *Itogi Nauki i Techniki, Mol. Biol.,* 19, 7, 1982.

52. **Payvar, F., Wrange, O., Carlstedt-Duke, J., Okret, S., Gustafsson, J.-O., and Yamamoto, K. R.,** Purified glucocorticoid receptors bind selectively in vitro to a cloned DNA fragment whose transcription is regulated by glucocorticoids in vivo, *Proc. Natl. Acad. Sci. USA,* 78, 6628, 1981.

53. **Groner, B., Kennedy, N., Skrach, P., Hynes, N. E., and Pouta, H.,** DNA sequences involved in the regulation of gene expression by glucocorticoid hormones, *Biochim. Biophys. Acta,* 781, 1, 1984.

54. **Mueller, G. C.,** Steroid hormone action: comments on the nature of the problem, in *Gene Regulation of Steroid Hormone,* Roy, A. K. and Clark, J. H., Eds., Springer-Verlag, New York, 1980.

55. **Hiremoth, S. T., Maciewiec, R. A., and Wang, T. Y.,** The loosely bound non-histone chromosomal proteins of rat prostate in androgen action, *Biochim. Biophys. Acta,* 653, 130, 1981.

56. **Spelsberg, T. C., Lifflefield, B. A., Seelke, R., Dani, G. M., Toyoda, H., Boyd-Leinen, P., Thrall, C., and Kon, O. L.,** Role of specific chromosomal proteins and DNA sequences in the nuclear binding sites for steroid receptors, *Prog. Horm. Res.,* 39, 463, 1983.

57. **Hiremath, S. T., Loor, R. M., and Wang, T. Y.,** Isolation of an androgen acceptor from salt extract of rat prostatic chromatin, *Biochem. Biophys. Res. Commun.,* 97, 981, 1980.

58. **Davies, P.,** Extraction of androgen-receptor complexes from regions of rat ventral prostate nuclei sensitive or resistant to nucleases, *J. Endocrinol.,* 99, 51, 1983.

59. **Lim, S. Y. and Ohno, S.,** The binding of androgen receptor to DNA and RNA, *Biochim. Biophys. Acta,* 654, 181, 1981.

60. **Tata, J. R.,** Do steroid receptors recognize DNA sequences?, *Nature,* 298, 707, 1982.

61. **Socher, S. H., Krall, J. F., Jaffe, E., and O'Malley, B. N.,** Distribution of binding sites for the progesterone receptor within chick oviduct chromatin, *Endocrinology,* 99, 891, 1976.

62. **Yamomoto, K. R., Gehring, U., Stampper, M. R., and Sibley, C. H.,** Genetic approaches to steroid hormone action, *Rec. Prog. Horm. Res.,* 32, 3, 1976.

63. **Spelsberg, T. C., Pikler, G. M., and Webster, R. A.,** Progesterone binding to hen oviduct genome: specific versus non-specific binding, *Science,* 194, 197, 1976.

64. **Williams, D. and Gorski, J.,** Kinetic and equilibrium analysis of estradiol in uterus: a model of binding-site distribution in uterine cells, *Proc. Natl. Acad. Sci. USA,* 69, 3464, 1972.

65. **Chomness, G. C., Lenning, A. W., and McGuire, W. L.,** Estrogen receptor binding to isolated nuclei. A nonsaturable process, *Biochemistry,* 13, 327, 1974.

66. **Yamomoto, K. R. and Alberts, B. M.,** On the specificity of the binding of the estradiol receptor protein to deoxyribonucleic acid, *J. Biol. Chem.,* 249, 7076, 1974.

67. **Thanki, K. H., Beach, T. A., and Dickerman, H. W.,** Selective binding of mouse estradiol receptor complexes to oligo (dT)-cellulose, *J. Biol. Chem.,* 253, 7744, 1978.

68. **Yamomoto, K. R. and Alberts, B. M.,** Steroid receptors: elements for modulation of eukaryotic transcription, *Annu. Rev. Biochem.,* 45, 721, 1976.

69. **Compton, J. C., Schrader, W. T., and O'Malley,** DNA sequence preference of the progesterone receptor, *Proc. Natl. Acad. Sci. USA,* 80, 16, 1983.

70. **Mulhivil, E. R., Pennec, J. P., and Chambon, P.,** Chicken oviduct progesterone receptor: location of specific regions of high-affinity binding in cloned DNA fragment of hormone-responsive genes, *Cell,* 28, 621, 1982.

71. **Rossind, G. P. and Lino, S.,** Intracellular interaction, reaction and dynamic status of prostate androgen receptors, *Biochem. J.,* 208, 383, 1982.

72. **Liao, S., Smyth, S., Tymoczko, J. L., Rossini, G. P., Chen, C., and Hiipakka, R. A.,** RNA-dependent release of androgen and other steroid receptor complexes from DNA, *J. Biol. Chem.,* 155, 5545, 1980.

73. **Lin, S. and Ohno, S.,** The interaction of androgen receptor with poly(A)-containing RNA and polyribonucleotides, *Eur. J. Biochem.,* 124, 283, 1982.

74. **Auricchio, F., Migliaccio, A., Castoria, G.,** Dephosphorylation of oestradiol nuclear receptor in vitro, *Biochem. J.,* 198, 199, 1981.

75. **Steel, R. V., Wilson, M. J., Ahmed, K., and Veneziale, C. M.,** Protein phosphatase activity on nuclear envelope from seminal vesicle epithelium, *Cell Mol. Biol.,* 28, 559, 1982.

76. **Lefebyre, Y. A. and Novosad, Z.,** Binding of androgens to a nuclear-envelope fraction from the rat ventral prostate, *Biochem. J.,* 186, 641, 1980.

77. **Kline, L. D., Lefebyre, Y. A., and Lefebyre, F. A. T.,** Uptake of androgens by intact and detergent-treated nuclei from ventral prostate, *J. Steroid Biochem.,* 14, 855, 1981.

78. **Barrack, E. R. and Coffrey, D. S.,** The role of the nuclear matrix in steroid hormone action, *Biochem. Actions Horm.,* 10, 23, 1983.

79. **Barrack, E. R.,** The nuclear matrix of the prostate contains acceptor sites for androgen receptors, *Endocrinology,* 113, 430, 1983.

80. **Epperly, M., Donofrio, J., Barham, S. S., and Veneziale, C. M.,** Nuclear protein matrix of seminal vesicle epithelium, *J. Steroid Biochem.,* 20, 691, 1984.

81. **Rennie, P. S., Bruchovsky, N., and Cheng, H.,** Isolation of 38 androgen receptors from salt-resistant fractions and nuclear matrixes of prostatic nuclei after mild trypsin digestion, *J. Biol. Chem.,* 258, 7623, 1983.

82. **Vollmer, G., Haase, A., and Eisele, K.,** Androgen receptor complex binding in murine skeletal muscle nuclei, *Biochem. Biophys. Res. Commun.,* 105, 1554, 1982.

83. **Stepanov, M. G. and Feldcoren, B. I.,** Androgen binding by skeletal muscles nuclei, *Bull. Exp. Biol. Med. (USSR),* 97, 606, 1984.

84. **Minguell, J. and Valladares, L.,** Molecular aspects on the mechanism of action of testosterone in rat bone marrow cells, *J. Steroid Biochem.,* 5, 649, 1974.

85. **Valladared, L. and Minguell, J.,** Characterization of a nuclear receptor for testosterone in rat bone marrow, *Steroids,* 25, 13, 1975.

86. **Liao, S., Liang, T., Shao, T. C., and Tymoczko, J. L.,** Androgen receptor cycling in prostate cells, *Adv. Exp. Med. Biol.,* 36, 232, 1973.

87. **Liao, S., Liang, T., and Tymoczko, J. L.,** Ribonucleoprotein binding of steroid "receptor" complexes, *Nature,* 241, 311, 1973.

88. **Walters, M. R. and Clark, J. H.,** Cytosol and nuclear compartmentalization of progesterone receptors of the rat uterus, *Endocrinology,* 103, 601, 1978.

89. **Baudendistel, L. J., Ruh, M. F., Nadel, E. M., and Ruh, T. S.,** Cytoplasmic oestrogen receptor replenishment: oestrogens versus antioestrogens, *Acta Endocrinol.,* 89, 599, 1978.

90. **Migliaccio, A., Lastoria, S., Moncharmont, B., Rotondi, A., and Auricchio, F.,** Phosphorylation of calf uterum 17β-estradiol receptor by endogenus Ca^{2+}-stimulated kinase activating the hormone binding of the receptor, *Biochem. Biophys. Res. Commun.,* 109, 1002, 1982.

91. **Auricchio, A., Migliaccio, A., Castaria, G., Rotondi, A., and Lastoria, S.,** Direct evidence of in vitro phosphorylation-dephosphorylation of the estradiol-17β, *J. Steroid Biochem.,* 20, 31, 1984.

92. **Miller, S. B. and Toft, D. O.,** Requirement for activation in the binding of progesterone receptor to ATP-sepharose, *Biochemistry,* 17, 173, 1978.

93. **Moudgil, V. K.,** Interaction of nucleotides with steroid hormone receptors, in *Molecular Mechanism of Steroid Hormone Action,* Moudgil, V. K., Ed., Walter de Gruyter, Berlin, 1985.

94. **Nemoto, T., Ohara-Nemoto, Y., Sato, N., Kyakumoto, S., and Oto, M.,** Characterization of nontransformed and transformed androgen receptor from rat submandibular gland, *Biochim. Biophys. Acta,* 839, 249, 1985.

95. **Okamoto, K., Ishohashi, F., Horiuchi, M., and Sakamoto, V.,** Three forms of macromol-

ecular translocation inhibitor of the nuclear binding of activated receptor-glucocorticoid complex and their interaction with ATP, *Biochem. Biophys. Res. Commun.,* 108, 1655, 1982.

96. **Okamoto, K., Ishohashi, F., Horiuchi, M., and Sakamoto, V.,** An ATP-stimulated factor that enhances the nuclear binding of activated receptor-glucocorticoid complex, *Biochem. Biophys. Res. Commun.,* 121, 940, 1984.

97. **Logeat, F., Le Cunff, M., Pomphila, R., and Milgrom, E.,** The nuclear-bound form of the progesterone receptor is generated through a hormone-dependent phosphorylation, *Biochem. Biophys. Res. Commun.,* 131, 426, 1985.

98. **Shoefer, E., Chock, P. B., and Stadtman, E. R.,** Regulation through phosphorylation/dephosphorylation cascade systems, *J. Biol. Chem.,* 25, 12252, 1984.

99. **Shoefer, E., Chock, P. B., Stadtman, E. R.,** Energy consumption in a cyclic phosphorylation/dephosphorylation cascade, *J. Biol. Chem.,* 259, 12260, 1984.

100. **King, W. S. and Greene, G. L.,** Monoclonal antibodies localize oestrogen receptor in the nuclei of target cells, *Nature,* 307, 745, 1984.

101. **Welshons, W. V., Lieberman, M. E., and Grski, J.,** Nuclear localization of unoccupied oestrogen receptors, *Nature,* 307, 347, 1984.

102. **Press, M. F., Holt, S. A., Hebrest, A. L., and Greene, G. L.,** Immunocytochemical identification of estrogen receptor in ovarian carcinomas, *Lab. Invest.,* 53, 349, 1985.

103. **King, R. J. B.,** Enlightenment and confusion over steroid hormone receptors, *Nature,* 312, 701, 1982.

104. **Greene, G. L. and King, W. S.,** Greene and King reply, *Nature,* 317, 88, 1985.

105. **Gorski, J.,** Gorski replies, *Nature,* 317, 89, 1985.

106. **Shull, S. D., Welshons, W. V., Lieberman, M. E., and Gorski, S.,** The rat pituitary estrogen receptor: role of the nuclear receptor in the regulation of transcription of the prolactin gene and the nuclear localization of the unoccupied receptor, in, *Molecular Mechanism of Steroid Hormone Action,* Moudgil, V. K., Ed., Walter de Gruyter, Berlin, 1985.

107. **Milgrom, E. and Atger, M.,** Receptor translation inhibitor and apparent saturability of the nuclear acceptor, *J. Steroid Biochem.,* 6, 487, 1975.

108. **MacDonald, R. G. and Leavitt, W. W.,** Reduced sulphydryl groups are required for activation of uterine progesterone receptor, *J. Biol. Chem.,* 257, 311, 1982.

109. **Liao, S., Chen, C., and Huang, I. J.,** Prostate α-protein, *J. Biol. Chem.,* 257, 122, 1982.

110. **Brinkmann, A. O., Lindh, L. M., and Breedveld, D. J.,** Cyproterone acetate prevents translocation of the androgen receptor in the rat prostate, *Mol. Cell. Endocrinol.,* 32, 117, 1983.

111. **Shyr, C. J. and Liao, S.,** Protein factor that inhibits binding and promotes release of androgen-receptor complex from nuclear chromatin, *Proc. Natl. Sci. USA,* 75, 5969, 1978.

112. **Mulder, E., Vrij, A. A., and Brinkmann, A. O.,** DNA and ribonucleotide binding characteristics of two forms of the androgen receptor from rat prostate, *Biochem. Biophys. Res. Commun.,* 114, 1147, 1983.

Chapter 5

MOLECULAR MECHANISMS OF AAS ACTION

Today only the first step in studying the mechanism of AAS action has been taken. However, by now there can be no doubt that the receptors appear to be one of the main links in the mechanism which ensures the realization of the hormonal signal at the level of gene expression. Experimental data on the high degree of correlation between the presence of receptors and the reactivation of tissues and between hormone affinity for androgen receptors and its biological effectiveness are the basis for the hypothesis of the important role of receptors in the realization of AAS hormonal effects. Summing up the basic alterations in metabolism which are observed at early stages of AAS action, one could note the following events:

1. Rapid stimulation of the activity of nuclear RNA polymerases and RNA synthesis.
2. Ability of RNA, extracted from the cells and worked up with steroid hormones, to cause some hormonal responses in hormone deficient cells.
3. Prevention of the effect of steroids by inhibitors of RNA and protein synthesis.
4. Induction of proteins including enzymes.

The cardinal successes in studying the mechanism of AAS action were achieved with target organ work, and primarily with sex tissues. The first investigations using AAS already showed that these hormones, like natural androgens (testosterone, dihydrotestosterone), caused retardative biological effects. The action from the moment of AAS injection into an organism to the appearance of maximum hormonal effect takes a long period of time. This factor probably decided, to some extent, the choice of criteria for the estimation of AAS action. They were basically determined by means of morphological character-istics of additional male sex organs.[1] It turned out that all the AAS used in the experiments possessed, to a greater or lesser degree, an androgenic activity which was distinctly revealed in special tests. Therefore, a comparative analysis of the action of 13 AAS on the change of comb size in chicks was carried out. It was established that all the AAS investigated exhibited an androgenic activity which may change from one steroid to another in sufficiently large quantities and which is conditioned by the presence of separate functional groups in the structure of the hormone.[2] A comparison of the action of 22 AAS demonstrated the changes that occur in prostate and seminal vesicle weight in rats, which depended on the dose and structure of the steroid used.[3] It turned out that in order to show distinct changes in prostate and seminal vesicle weight, it was necessary to use much larger doses than for the change of m.l.a. weight.[4] As Figure 16 shows, a prolonged methandrostenolone injection (0.3 mg/kg) into rats leads to

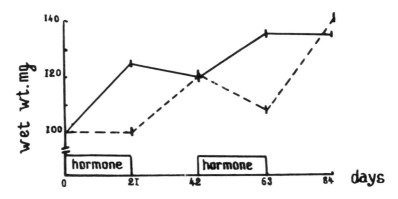

FIGURE 16.   Effect of methandrostenolone on rat prostate weight. — Without hormone, - - with hormone.

an inhibition of endocrine gland function and subsequent growth retardation. On the 21st day after AAS injection, an increase in citric acid content in seminal vesicles and ventral prostate was seen, as well as the retardation of the growth of these organs. After cessation of AAS injection, the weight of the endocrine glands and their function gradually returned to their normal level. A repeated AAS injection again led to retardation of the development of the endocrine glands and their function and was marked by a reduction in weight and a decrease in the content of citric acid and the quantity of liquid secreted. Three weeks after ceasing AAS injections, a gradual reduction of sex gland function was observed, as well as an increase in weight. Therefore, prolonged AAS use was associated with essential alterations in the function of rat sex glands and led to the inhibition of their development.[5] The discovery of specific biochemical indices (citric acid, fructose, polyamines) characterizing androgen action in prostate led to the development using direct estimation of the metabolic state of the organ instead of simply using morphological signs. Injection of androgens and AAS into an organism causes the induction of a large number of enzymes in the prostate and other male sex organs and is localized in various subcell components. Among them one can mention RNA polymerase of nuclei, cytochrome oxidase of mitochondria, β-glucuronidase of lysosome, aldolase of cytoplasm, and ATPase of microsome. These enzymes and a number of others are activated under the influence of androgens and AAS.[6] The results of studying protein synthesis in rat prostate showed that this process was under the control of androgens. The change of androgen concentration or their removal has a considerable effect on the synthesis of proteins. In addition, stimulation of protein synthesis by androgens proved to be a very slow process which can proceed for many hours. A number of works have investigated the influence of androgens on the synthesis and protein metabolism of endoplasmic membranes of prostate.[7,8] It has been shown that protein synthesis occurs within the fraction of heavy membranes of the endoplasmic reticulum. The movement of ^{14}C-choline into phospholipids in these membranes is also regulated by androgens. The membranes of other prostate-like secretary organs are characterized by a rapid metabolism and a high rate of turnover of all components. By examining the mechanisms of androgen regulator action on the processes of protein synthesis in the prostate, one can distinguish several stages where the effect of these steroids has been experimentally demonstrated: the synthesis of mRNA containing poly (A) at the 3′ end,[7] mRNA processing and modification in cytoplasm,[8] synthesis and assembly by means of polyribosome,[9] and the synthesis of aldolase and the regulation of its activity.[10,11] Without taking into consideration the control of protein and lipid synthesis, androgens actively participate in the regulation of a number of reactions of intracellular metabolism which are associated with the conversion of glucose and some amino acids. Thus, in the example of androgens and AAS action in the prostate, one can conclude that these steroid hormones actively participate in the preservation of the structure and the regulation of sex gland function. In comparison with the rapid progress of uncovering the mechanism of AAS metabolism in the prostate, there exists a considerable lag in investigations carried out in skeletal muscles.

As mentioned earlier, the first works investigating the mechanism of AAS action clearly showed their activated effect on the weight growth of various skeletal muscles which is associated with the retention of nitrogen and water in the organism.[1,12] Results of experiments on adult guinea pigs (both healthy and castrated), which were implantated with various AAS for a period of 30 days, showed that at the end of the time period there was an increase in body mass. Muscle mass increased in various groups under the influence of AAS and was dependent on the hormone dose. Estimation of the anabolic actions of 12 AAS demonstrated the influence of the position of separate functional groups. It turned out that the presence of a methyl group in position 17 of the steroid molecule considerably reduced anabolic activity.[13,14]

These results show an active participation of AAS in the process of protein synthesis in skeletal muscle and indicate the presence of several sites of steroid action. Cell free systems were used to objectively study the effect of AAS on separate stages of the synthesis of muscular proteins. It was quite natural to initially investigate transcription processes in muscle cells. The transcription process is carried out by RNA polymerases and their factors. In the cells of eukaryotes, there exist three different RNA polymerases: I, nucleolus polymerase ensuring the synthesis of ribosomal RNA predecessors; II, nucleoplasmatic RNA polymerase carrying out chromatin transcription in the form of heterogeneous nuclear RNA — the predecessors of all the mRNA forms; and III, the RNA polymerase synthesizing several short types of RNA including 5 S RNA and tRNA. Each of these enzymes transcribes a certain set of genes. RNA polymerase II transcribes thousands of different genes coding the proteins. RNA polymerase III transcribes a rather limited number of genes, and RNA polymerase I exclusively affects one kind of transcriptional unit, the gene of ribosomal RNA.[15] RNA polymerases represent compound complexes consisting of several subunits (β, β′, α and σ), each of which accomplish a certain function.[16] All three RNA polymerase complexes differ in the antibiotics that inhibit them. Cycloheximide inhibits the activity of RNA polymerase I while α-amanitin inhibits II and III. The process of RNA synthesis, catalyzed by RNA polymerase I and II, includes several stages: enzyme combination to DNA-matrix, synthesis initiation, elongation (an increase in the synthesized RNA chain), and termination (the completion of RNA synthesis). At the first stage the interaction of an enzyme with a promoter occurs where the selectivity and the binding strength of these components are due to the presence of the factor σ. It is only after combination with factor σ that RNA polymerase alters its conformation and turns into an active form which is able to accomplish the subsequent RNA synthesis. After completing the stage of initiation, the factor σ separates from the enzyme. The promoter consists of 40 to 50 pairs of nucleotides and is not transcribed by the enzyme. At subsequent stages of transcription, RNA synthesis occurs in the presence of substrates and cofactors. To evaluate the effect of AAS, the activity of nuclear RNA polymerase II was investigated at the stage of transcription. It turned out that a single injection of methylandrostanediol into rats caused a considerable increase in enzyme activity (Table 10). Another AAS — methandienone — also increases enzyme activity, but to a lesser degree. It should be noted that these results were obtained in a cell free system *in vitro* and in the presence of ammonium sulfate, which caused chromatin dissociation and released DNA from histones. Under these conditions, the acceleration of transcription testifies to a stimulating effect of AAS on enzyme activity. Thus, the role of AAS in regulation in the stage of transcription at the level of RNA polymerase II was experimentally demonstrated.

From the results arose the question, "How is the effect of AAS manifested during physical activity?"

Some experiments were carried out on a model system which has been used in our laboratory for studying nuclear-plasmatic relations in skeletal muscles. The uniqueness of this system consists of adding cytoplasm extract to homologous nuclei obtained from animal skeletal muscles under diverse conditions.

As Table 11 shows, the addition of cytoplasmic extract obtained from exer-

TABLE 10
Nuclear RNA Polymerase Activity of Rat
Skeletal Muscle After AAS Injection

	RNA polymerase activity (pmol ^{3}H-UMP/mg DNA)	
Experimental conditions	Full system	Without $(NH_4)_2SO_4$
Without hormone	724 ± 34	516 ± 27
With methandienone	845 ± 32	836 ± 36
With methylandrostanediol	922 ± 68	575 ± 48

TABLE 11
Change of RNA Polymerase Activity in Model System with Nuclei and Cytoplasmic Extract of Skeletal Muscles Using AAS

Variants of model system	Hormone	RNA polymerase activity (pmol ^{3}H-UMP/mg DNA $\pm$ SD)
Nuclei-rest Cytoplasm-rest	Without hormone	1118 ± 43
Nuclei-rest Cytoplasm-exercise	Without hormone	885 ± 23
Nuclei-rest Cytoplasm-exercise	With methandienone	1091 ± 51
Nuclei-rest Cytoplasm-exercise	With methylandrostanediol	1168 ± 68

cised muscles (swimming for 15 min) of animals caused an inhibition of nuclear DNA, which is dependent on RNA polymerase activity, by 26%.

Injection of methandienone or methylandrostanediol into animals removed the inhibiting effect of skeletal muscle cytoplasm in working animals. In this case the enzyme activity was the same as at rest.

The findings obtained showed that AAS participated in the regulation of the transcription stage and increased the activity of nuclear RNA polymerase II in skeletal muscles. One may believe that in the process of enzyme activation, the critical moment is the steroid-receptor complex binding to chromatin acceptor sites. We also investigated the dependence of the activity of skeletal muscle RNA polymerase I on the time of AAS action. After a single injection of nandrolone-decanoate into rats, a considerable (to 58%) and steady (more than 4 days) increase in RNA polymerase I activity was observed. The data in Table 12 show that 14 hours after AAS injection, enzyme activity rose by 45% and in subsequent days it remained at that level.

It should be noted that a group of rapid turnover proteins can also take part in the regulation of rRNA synthesis. The inhibitor of protein synthesis, cyclo-heximide, was used for determining such proteins in rRNA transcription in skeletal muscle nuclei. It has been established that by the injection of cyclo-heximide into animals, the inhibition of RNA-synthesizing capability of skeletal muscle nuclei demonstrates a positive straight line relationship with time. It is characterized by the kinetics of a first-order reaction with a half-life period of rapid turnover proteins participating in the control of enzyme activity equal to 110 min.[18] Table 12 also gives data for determining the period of a protein half-life participating in the control of rRNA synthesis. It is very interesting that the increase in RNA synthesizing capability of skeletal muscle nuclei after AAS injection is accompanied by a rise in the half-life of the proteins participation in the control of RNA polymerase I activity. One can assume that the rise in activity

TABLE 12
Effect of Nandrolone-Decanoate on rRNA
Transcription of Skeletal Muscles

Time after injection (hr)	RNA polymerase activity (%)	Half-life period of fast turnover proteins (%)
0	100	100
14	145	135
72	158	150
96	148	—

of nuclear RNA polymerase I in skeletal muscle is accomplished primarily by means of control mechanisms involving the fraction of rapid turnover proteins of rRNA transcription and not by increasing the quantity of the enzyme. In subsequent functional investigations in order to reveal the role of rapid turnover proteins in the regulation of RNA transcription, we compared data on RNA polymerase activity of skeletal muscle nuclei with results of the determination of the half-life of the proteins.[19] Based on the results of previous investigations it was established that systematic AAS-nandrolone-decanoate injections (4 times) caused considerable stimulation of rRNA synthesis muscular tissue nuclei. The kinetics of the RNA polymerase reaction occurring in nuclei did not appreciably change and the time of completion of RNA synthesis was the same. These data testify to the increase in rRNA transcription due to the increase in the frequency of RNA polymerase initiation *in vivo*, which is manifested *in vitro* in a high RNA-synthesizing capability of skeletal muscle nuclei. The determination of the half-life of chromatin rapid turnover proteins shows that by injection of nandrolone-decanoate, the velocity of protein exchange essentially increased as well.[20] Thus, one may conclude that AAS participate in regulation of the synthesis of ribosomal RNA in skeletal muscle which is manifested in a rise in nuclear DNA-dependent RNA polymerase I activity and in a change in the half-life of transcriptional complex regulative proteins. One can believe that the process of RNA polymerase activation is also reflected by the synthesis of other RNA types. The increase in amino acids included in skeletal muscle proteins after AAS injection into an organism may be certain confirmation of such an assumption. As Figure 17 shows, after injection of methandienone into rats, ^{14}C-leucine in skeletal muscle protein is increased. Under the influence of AAS, the transport of amino acids to skeletal muscles rose, and an increase in ^{14}C-leucine content in myosin, myofibrillar and sarcoplasmic proteins occurred. While examining this increase of labeled amino acids in muscular proteins after AAS-methandienone injection, it should be noted that these data confirm the observations of the increase in the amount of actin and myosin in guinea pig muscle after injection of testosterone derivatives.[21]

An intensification of protein metabolism in skeletal muscle under the influ-

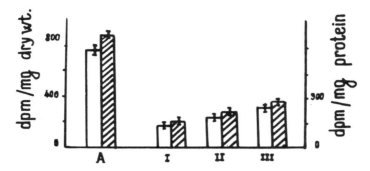

FIGURE 17. Effect of methandienone ▨ on transport (A) and ^{14}C-leucine incorporation into myosin (I), myofibrillar (II) and sarcoplasmic (III) protein of skeletal muscles.

ence of AAS is accompanied not only by an increase in synthesis of basic contractile proteins, that is actin and myosin, but to some extent it is reflected by the synthesis of separate enzymes. Thus, by injecting methandienone, the activity of several enzymes rises in rat skeletal muscles and is localized in various subcellular structures: nuclear DNA-dependent RNA polymerase,[20] mitochondrial cytochrome oxidase,[5] cytoplasmic aminotransferase.[22] It is necessary to note that this hormone, like other AAS, does not participate in the alteration of enzyme activity as a modulator. The influence of AAS on tissue enzymes occurs by means of a complicated chain of reactions participating in the process of protein biosynthesis. The effect of AAS is accomplished primarily via the mechanism of intensification which is involved with a quantitative change in mRNA synthesis and not with a qualitative modulation and a spectrum expansion of mRNA molecules which are synthesized anew. Thus, the induction of some enzymes may be considered to be one of the highly specific manifestations of AAS action in the organism. To confirm the validity of such a conclusion we cite the data where the induction of the enzymes occurs under the influence of AAS (Table 13). As can be seen these enzymes, where their activity changes under the influence of AAS action is of great significance for discovering the mechanism of enzyme induction.

In addition to skeletal muscle, liver, and kidneys, the induction of separate enzymes under the influence of AAS, and in particular aldolase, is clearly shown in sex organs.

Comparison of the changes in the activity of separate enzymes to the velocity of the exchange of separate metabolic cycles and to at last carbohydrate, lipid, and protein metabolism in skeletal muscle by AAS injection into the organism is similar in many respects to the anabolic phase of the process of muscular tissue adaptation to systematic physical exercise. A single muscular activity is known to cause some alterations of metabolism in skeletal muscles. Under the influence of systematic muscular activity, these alterations in metabolism accumulate and

TABLE 13
Enzymes Increasing Activity Under
AAS Influence

Tissue	Enzyme	Ref.
Skeletal	Aminotransferases	13, 22
muscles	Pyruvate kinase	23
	Succinate dehydrogenase	12
	Cytochrome c oxidase	5, 24
	β-Glucuronidase	24
	Arylsulphatase	24
	RNA polymerase I and II	18, 20
Liver	Tyrosine aminotransferase	25
	Fumarase	25

when summed up can lead to considerable functional and structural reconstructions in muscular tissue.[29] There exist essential morphological and biochemical differences between trained and untrained skeletal muscle.[30,31] Biochemical alterations occurring in skeletal muscle under the influence of their systematic function are specific enough and dependent on the character of the physical exercise used. Thus, strength physical exercises are first accompanied by some structural changes in contractile proteins. They lead to the largest increase in muscular mass and ATPase activity. The speed at which physical exercise is performed is associated more with the process of ATP anaerobic production and oxidative phosphorylation. Prolonged physical exercises are performed under the conditions of metabolic steady state and principally exert influence on the development of the processes of ATP aerobic resynthesis accompanied by a rise in oxidative enzyme activity.

According to the character of alterations caused by the metabolism of skeletal muscles, a number of common traits may be observed in the action of AAS and physical loads. Generally they can be represented as an active effect on the process of protein synthesis. A comparison of separate indices of metabolism is by analogy justified up to a certain limit, but it does not help to explain the molecular mechanism of action of these two factors. Therefore, experiments with simultaneous action on AAS skeletal muscle and systematic function are needed. In our laboratory we carried out a prolonged experiment where rats performed intensive strength exercises for 84 days and were injected with 0.3 mg/kg of methandienone (2 courses, each for 21 days). The findings demonstrated an intensification of anabolic processes and the stimulation of basic metabolic pathways ensuring an increase in muscular protein synthesis.[5,22] We also investigated the velocity at which ^{14}C-orotic acid was incorporated into RNA fractions, ^{14}C-leucine into muscular proteins and amino acids, as well as the activity of cytochrome oxidase and aspartate aminotransferase and the content of glycogen, ATP, CP and lactic acid in skeletal muscle. The findings showed that the functional activity of skeletal muscle determined the intensity of the development of anabolic processes following exercise. It is of considerable importance for the manifestation of hormone action that the dose exceed a certain threshold value. Our experiments showed an increase in muscular tissue radioactivity, by injection of ^{14}C-leucine and ^{14}C-orotic acid into the animals which had received methandienone following exercise, which testifies to the hormone effect on the mechanism of substance transport regulation to skeletal muscles. As stated above, AAS injection into an organism causes a rise in DNA-dependent RNA polymerase I activity in skeletal muscle.[18] It seems reasonable to hypothesize that AAS use during systematic muscular activity is also reflected by this enzyme activity. The data obtained on the rise of RNA polymerase I activity in the nuclei of rat skeletal muscle subjected to exercise training confirms this supposition (Table 14). One can see that exercise training induces a rise in enzyme activity by 47%. After four injections of nandrolone-decanoate during the training process, RNA polymerase activity rose by 93% in comparison with the control.[19] The kinetics of this reaction confirmed the fact that the increase in RNA synthesis in skeletal muscle was associated with a rise in RNA polymerase activity.[20] A rise in the activity of cytochrome-C oxidase and aspartate aminotransferase parallel with the acceleration of the incorporation of ^{14}C-leucine into myofibrillar and sarcoplasmic proteins testifies to the activation of protein synthesis processes in muscle under the influence of AAS.

The data obtained give an indication of the presence of many factors that can determine the development of methandienone anabolic action in skeletal muscle by an intensive muscular activity. One may consider that the intensification of skeletal muscle metabolism during systematic physical activity increases the sensitivity of muscular tissue to methandienone, and the threshold values of hormone effective doses prove to be lower than those under the usual regime.

This was confirmed by the experiments that studied AAS reception in the skeletal muscle of exercise trained animals (Table 15).

One can see that systematic muscular activity causes an increase in androgen reception in rat skeletal muscle cytoplasm.[20] It may lead to the intensification of RNA synthesis in muscle even if the level of androgens in the blood does not

TABLE 14
Effect of Training and Nandrolone-Decanoate on Nuclear RNA Polymerase Activity of Rat Skeletal Muscles

Experimental conditions	pmol ^{3}H-UMP/mg DNA $\pm$ SD
Control	73 ± 5
Training	107 ± 9
Training with nandrolone-decanoate	141 ± 9

TABLE 15
Effect of Training and Nandrolone-Decanoate
on Androgen Reception in Skeletal Muscle
Cytoplasm

Experimental conditions	dpm/mg protein ± SD
Control	108 ± 8
Training	185 ± 16
Training with nandrolone-decanoate	146 ± 11

change. The injection of nandrolone-decanoate during training also causes an increase in androgen reception, however on a smaller scale in comparison with actual training. Subsequent experiments have determined that 19-nortestosterone injection into animals which have performed systematic speed-strength exercises caused an increase in nuclear androgen receptor content in skeletal muscles as well.[32] One can conclude that AAS selectively induce the synthesis of their own receptor proteins in muscle based on the rise in androgen receptor concentration in cytoplasm and skeletal muscle nuclei. Thus, the intensification of intracellular skeletal muscle metabolism during a systematic function and AAS exert a synergistic action on the process of protein synthesis. This is reflected by not only an increase in the amount of contractile and enzyme proteins, but also in the inductive synthesis of proper androgen receptor proteins. Evidently, AAS exert a regulating influence on the process of hormone reception in which they are able to essentially control all stages of the receptor cycle including the stage of nuclear binding. Hence, the amount of androgen receptors in muscular tissue may change under the influence of systematic physical activities and AAS, which also changes the sensitivity of this tissue towards AAS.

The findings confirm published data on the ability of isometric training and nandrolone-decanoate injection.[33] This work also shows that isometric training itself exerts a diverse action on the metabolism of fast- and slow-twitch skeletal muscle. The gender of the animal is of great importance, too. After AAS injection, alterations in the energy metabolism of skeletal muscle are expressed more distinctly in males than in females.[34] It should also be noted that AAS anabolic action cannot always be demonstrated in experiments where the animals have been physically trained. In an experiment using rats, the animals were run on a treadmill in a series of short exercise bouts: 6 sec running, 6 sec rest, speed — 48 m/min, for a total of 6 series per day for 90 days. For 48 days the animals were injected with methandienone (0.35 mg/kg of weight a day). It was observed that under the influence of the training, the strength of skeletal muscles and general physical endurance increased. However, there were no differences in these and other biochemical indices in the animals trained while taking methandienone and the controls. The injection of methandienone led to an appreciable decrease in the level of luteinizing hormone in the blood of trained and untrained animals.[36]

The participation of AAS in metabolic regulation is not limited to sex organs and skeletal muscles. These steroid hormones actively regulate metabolism in other various organs and tissues of an organism.[13,37] The plurality of AAS hormonal effects which regulate separate reactions of carbohydrate,[38] lipid, and protein metabolism should be noted. By estimating the AAS anabolic action, the major effect is on the process of protein synthesis; however, these steroid hormones also considerably intensify lipid metabolism in the organism. AAS regulates the activity of separate enzyme reactions accelerating the oxidation of fatty acids. It should be taken into consideration that in addition to such diverse positive effects, the systematic use of AAS leads to a disturbance in the function of the organism's endocrine system. First of all, it alters the content of androgenous androgens themselves (luteinizing and follicle stimulating hormones, estrogens and a number of other hormones of steroid nature). A sharp inhibition of testosterone synthesis in Leydig cells is one of the most striking examples of such endocrine alterations which is associated with the presence of AAS. The basic enzymes responsible for testosterone synthesis in mammals are concentrated in endoplasmatic reticulum and mitochondria of Leydig cells.[39-41]

Attempts were made to bind the alterations in the level of testosterone secretion with those of ultrastructure and Leydig cell volume. It turned out that the alteration of testosterone secretion was closely associated with only one morphological index of these cells, the volume of smooth endoplasmic reticulum.[42,43] By injecting gonadotrophin into an organism, growth of smooth endoplasmic reticulum occurs and the amount of testosterone synthesized increases.[44] Conversely, by injecting AAS, some morphological alterations occur that lead to the diminution of smooth endoplasmic reticulum and the decrease of testosterone synthesis. The inhibition of testosterone synthesis is accompanied, in turn, by a change in concentration of this hormone in other androgen-dependent tissues. The change of androgen concentration was clearly demonstrated in the experiments which used a systematic method of training animals (Table 16).

The use of AAS nandrolone-phenylpropionate during such training regimens (1 mg/kg of mass/day, 8 times for 28-day training cycle) led to a decrease in the level of testosterone in blood, skeletal muscle and heart muscle. This phenomenon was demonstrated in experiments on animals of different gender and was linked with the inhibition of androgen synthesis by the use of AAS. A possible mechanism regulating the level of androgen in tissue is associated with the presence of androgen receptors, which prove to be occupied chiefly by AAS and their metabolites. It excludes the androgen hormones from the receptor sphere and, according to the mechanism of reverse bond, it inhibits the processes of their synthesis.

TABLE 16
Testosterone Content in Rat Organs
(pg/g wet wt ± SD)

Tissue or fluid	Nontrained	Trained	Trained with hormone taking
Blood	118.0 ± 22.7	64.0 ± 7.8	73.0 ± 5.3
Skeletal muscles	200.0 ± 34.3	100.6 ± 12.6	37.9 ± 5.8
Heart	235.0 ± 26.9	127.0 ± 19.5	64.4 ± 6.3

The ability of AAS to stimulate and regulate metabolism in tissues with various functional trends shows that the mechanism of their action varies in different tissues. It should be noted that the process of a hormonal signal pass (the idea of an obligatory AAS interaction with receptor proteins) does not always exactly correspond with such a mechanism. As the investigation of the binding specificity of 12 AAS by androgen receptors in rabbit and rat skeletal muscles[45] showed, essential differences between separate hormones were shown even in such a small group of steroids. The results showed that some AAS are very weakly bound to TEBG and therefore the existence of a specific transport protein remains open to debate, although their transport to target organs may apparently occur with the participation of blood albumins. There are also such AAS which weakly interact with androgen receptors of skeletal muscle but are also intensively bound to similar prostate receptors. There are also AAS which cannot interact with receptor proteins. Such a diverse character of AAS interaction with receptor proteins of skeletal muscle leads us to assume the presence of an alternative pathway of AAS action. Another approach to discover the mechanism of AAS action in skeletal muscle has been planned. Experiments on myoblast culture of rats show that trenbolone-acetate and testosterone influence the rate of muscular protein turnover only through the specific growth factors somatomedin and somatotropin.[46] In all probability, the action of AAS in muscles may be transferred through other hormones which regulate the processes of protein biosynthesis. According to all available data, outside of some positive effects of AAS on the processes of protein synthesis, these steroids may inhibit the activity of proteolytic enzymes. The reduction in the activity of cathepsin D in rat skeletal muscle after trenbolone-acetate injection leads to the end of muscular growth.[47] It was suggested that AAS reduced the rate of protein degradation, and it is this mechanism that is the basis of the anabolic action of these hormones. It is necessary to emphasize that although the investigations are methodologically sound, the results are somewhat relative. This can be explained by the fact that there is no direct experimental proof of the participation of AAS as a modulator of certain enzymes. Most likely, to the contrary, the idea about the pass of a hormonal signal by steroids to a target organ through the change of gene expression remains a dominating hypothesis. AAS action in target organs is directed to regulation of the synthesis of various proteins including enzymes. The realization of AAS action may be accomplished through the spectrum of hormones that specifically participate in the regulation of metabolism in target organs including skeletal muscle. A distinctive AAS feature lies in the fact that these steroid hormones act intracellularly and, in the first stages, they do not interact directly with the system of cyclic nucleotides. Through cellular membranes, passing the system of specific carriers, free AAS transport gives the impression of a certain autonomy, the isolation of AAS from other hormones. However, as the hormone approaches its ultimate goal, chromatin, it proves to be closely associated with many regulated processes of intracellular metabolism. Such an interaction occurs through the system of cyclic nucleotides, cAMP and cGMP and a group of enzymes through which the hormonal signal passes. The activity of these systems is tightly associated with the metabolism of calcium in the cell which in turn participates in the regulation of cyclic AMP-dependent and cyclic GMP-dependent protein kinases. The protein kinases may phosphorylate a considerable amount of chromatin proteins and participate in their modification. A successive cascade of reactions leads to the regulation of chromatin matrix activity. After the discovery of a system of intracellular metabolic regulations, with the participation of cyclic nucleotides, some attempts were made to determine their effect on the action of steroid hormones, in particular androgens. There also appeared those investigations that studied the effect of androgens on the system of enzymes linked with cyclic AMP metabolism. It should be noted that these initial investigations did not yield any significant results and the participation of cAMP in the regulation of androgen metabolism was primarily associated with the enzymes ensuring the synthesis of androgens in the reproductive glands. More evidence was obtained with the study of the influence of androgens on the enzymes associated with metabolism and level of cAMP in tissues. The content of cyclic nucleotides is closely connected with the activity of adenylate cyclases, the enzymes which ensure the synthesis of these substances, and phosphodiesterase enzymes which participate in their degradation. The maintenance of dynamic equilibrium in the reaction rates of these enzymes ensures a certain level of cyclic nucleotide in the cell. If the activity of these enzymes changes, the content of nucleotides will change as well.

Ascertainment of the fact that not only calmodulin but also other heat-resistant, calcium-dependent proteins (found in the heart, skeletal muscles, kidneys, and brain) can activate an enzyme proved to be essential in the regulation of phosphodiesterase activity. The phosphodiesterase activity in most tissues is sufficiently high; therefore the concentration of cAMP usually falls to basal values soon after hormonal stimulation has occurred. In addition to the proteins being able to activate enzymes, the proteins which inhibit phosphodiesterase were also revealed. A detailed study of the mechanism of action of phosphodiesterase heat-resistant inhibitor at different stages in the development of an organism established a close connection with the level of androgens in blood. The rise in testosterone concentration in blood caused the reduction of phosphodiesterase activity in reproductive glands, i.e., the change of androgen concentration in blood is reflected by the activity of an enzyme hydrolyzing cyclic nucleotides in the cell. The results showed that the inhibitor of phospho-diesterase activity was under the control of androgens.[48] Through a chain of successive reactions, testosterone and dihydrotestosterone affected the activation of certain sites of a genome which are associated with the synthesis of phosphodiesterase inhibitor. The rise of androgen concentration in blood leads to a reduction in phosphodiesterase activity and raises the concentration of cyclic AMP. This explains the rather high levels of cAMP in androgen-dependent tissues.[49] Thus, a regulative role of androgens in the change of intracellular concentrations of cyclic nucleotides was demonstrated.[50]

Injection of AAS into an organism shows their participation in cyclic nucleotide intracellular concentration, which may also be accomplished with a subsequent inclusion of all the reactions controlled by cAMP. In this case one can talk about the interaction of AAS, calcium, and the systems of cyclic nucleotides in the regulation of intracellular processes.

Now let us consider some possible molecular mechanisms of the specific effect of AAS on metabolism in muscular tissues and the mechanisms of these regulatory processes.

All the principal stages of steroid interaction that are typical for the other target organs, primarily for androgens, may be seen by the effects of intracellular AAS in skeletal muscle. Therefore, any potential mechanism of AAS participation in the regulation of metabolism should include the description of well-known notions of the succession of events which involve androgens. The differences may be as subtle as the method of injection of AAS into the organism and blood.

A possible model of AAS participation in the control of genetic expression in skeletal muscle is based on experimental data obtained in the past few years.[51-53] In general the outine for this model does not differ from the notions which have been currently accepted (described in detail in Chapter 4). The principal stage of hormonal signal passing includes the interaction of AAS with transport protein and migration to skeletal muscle, the penetration of such a transport complex into the muscular cell and the interaction of hormone with a specific receptor protein, the activation of the hormone-receptor complex and its subsequent translocation to a nucleus, interaction with chromatin acceptor sites, the alteration of a transcription level of separate genes, the release of the hormone-receptor complex from chromatin, the hormone dissociation from the receptor, and the return of the latter to cytoplasm. In the end, this complicated chain of events leads to an intensification of the process of protein synthesis which has an effect on the intensification of growth processes and the development of target tissues (Figure 18).

The order of temporary events occurring in skeletal muscle after 19-nortestosterone injection is given in Table 17.[54]

At present, many of the problems remain unsolved and without satisfactory

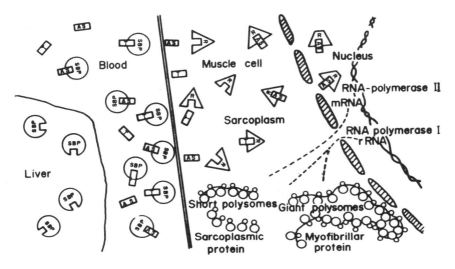

FIGURE 18. A possible model of AAS action in skeletal muscle.

TABLE 17
Temporary Distribution of Events
in Skeletal Muscle After
19-Nortestosterone Injection

Processes	Time (hr)
19-Nortestosterone binding to a receptor and transport to nucleus	0.1
mRNA synthesis	0.5
pRNA synthesis	2.0
Sarcoplasmic protein synthesis	5.0
Myofibrillar protein synthesis	10.0

explanation. The description of the events that occur during the interaction of a hormone-receptor complex with chromatin is considered to be one of the most complicated questions. What is the signal for the binding of a hormone-receptor complex to regulated DNA fragments of separate genes? The specificity of steroid hormone action is due to a specific activation of certain genes. It may be determined by the existence of specific acceptor sites in chromatin which, with a high affinity, selectively bind hormone-receptor complexes. These complexes control certain genome sites which are of great importance for hormone action.

The results of investigations that have studied the interaction between hormone-receptor complexes and chromatin have provided convincing evidence of the presence of such acceptor sites and testify to the ability of steroid hormones to selectively increase the production of specific enzymes or proteins in androgen-dependent tissues. Regarding the possible mechanisms of selective hormone effects, the hypothesis that has been suggested in this review seems to be attractive and convincing.[55] In the author's opinion, the principle of reaction specificity is the basis of the selectivity of hormone-receptor complex interaction with chromatin. A large amount of chromatin locuses permitting the binding of hormone-receptor complexes are supposed to contain separate regulated locuses, the interaction with which is of decisive significance for hormonal reaction developing. The development of a hypothesis involving diverse mechanisms of hormonal reaction regulation at the level of chromatin has been gaining acceptance. One of them ensures the possibility of the transcription of hormone-specific genome sites. The second leads to a general destabilization of chromatin structure as the result of a hormone-receptor complex binding to it. A high affinity of receptors for chromatin acceptor sites ensures the saturation of a genome at a very low concentration of receptor complexes.

Quantitative regulation of the transcription of hormone-dependent genome sites depends on the activity of the second mechanism. It is dependent on the concentration of hormone-receptor complexes in the nucleus.[56,57]

There exist other notions about the character of hormone-receptor complex interaction with specific DNA sequences which lead to the activation of specific genes.[58,59]

The regulation of a molecular mechanism of AAS interaction with proteins in muscular tissue includes several successive stages during which the change in concentration of the hormone itself, or the substance interacting with it, is reflected by the specific physiological effect of the hormone. Intracellular AAS binding by transport proteins in blood may be considered to be the first stage of the regulation. In the target cell itself there are no less than six stages in which the regulatory mechanism is possible:

1. AAS binding to a receptor in the cytoplasm;
2. Hormone-receptor complex translocation to the nucleus;
3. Hormone-receptor complex binding to nonhistone proteins of chromatin;
4. Hormone-receptor complex release from chromatin;
5. Hormone-receptor complex dissociation in nucleus;
6. Biotransformation of AAS and its metabolites.

It should be noted that in reality there are many more possibilities for regulated effects. To examine only the third and fourth stages associated with the regulation of gene expression, the number of the spheres of application of regulated effects may reach 11.[60]

As Figure 19 shows, gene regulation is considered to be the process that not only includes transcription, but also the formation of mature mRNA, its transport to polysomes, and protein synthesis.

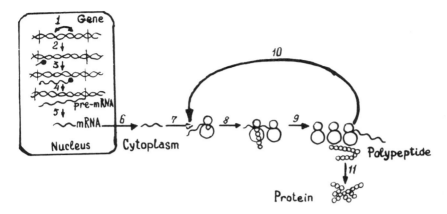

FIGURE 19. Possible levels on which gene regulation occurs.[61]

The following regulation sites are possible:

1. Genome reconstruction;
2. Transcription initiation;
3. Transcription elongation;
4. Transcription termination;
5. Pre-mRNA processing;
6. mRNA release to cytoplasm;
7. Translocation initiation;
8. Translocation elongation;
9. Translocation termination;
10. mRNA stability;
11. Peptide processing and protein self-assembling.

As experimental data show, regulation may be accomplished at all of these stages. However the basic factors were obtained for points 2 to 4 and 7 to 9, whereas information for the other points of possible regulatory effects is rare.[60]

By examining the processes of regulation at the level of transcription, it is necessary to note that many specialized (regulated) genes often appear to be multiple ones. Such a multiplicity was demonstrated for the genes which code specialized proteins (such as actin, tubulin) in skeletal muscle. The expression of specialized genes may be essentially altered due to an increase in their amount. These findings show that the hormones accomplish a quantitative and not qualitative regulation at the level of transcription. One can believe that AAS can also regulate quantitatively and change the transcription rate of certain specialized genes coding structural and contractile proteins at a muscular cell. Under the action of AAS, the transcription intensity increases, which leads to the saturation of polysomes by a large amount of mRNA. Additionally, the stabilization of mRNA molecules may also prolong the period of their turnover. Fom the moment of transcription and up to the combination to ribosomes, mRNA is combined with proteins which protect it from degradation. We have practically no information about a possible participation of steroid hormones, including AAS, in regulation at the level of transcription.

One can imagine that quantitative changes in the expression of certain, principally specialized, genes, which control the complicated multistage process of protein biosynthesis in a living cell, are the basis of the mechanism of AAS action.

REFERENCES

1. **Kochakian, C.,** Renotrophic-androgenic properties of orally administered androgens, *Proc. Soc. Exp. Biol.,* 80, 386, 1952.
2. **Boris, A. and Ng, Ch.,** Relative androgenic activities of some anabolic steroids as measured by chick-comb responses, *Steroids,* 9, 299, 1967.
3. **Dorfman, R. J. and Kincl, F. A.,** Relative potency of various steroids in an anabolic-androgenic assay using the castrated rat, *Endocrinology,* 72, 269, 1969.
4. **Boris, A., Stevenson, R. H., and Trimol, T.,** Comparative androgenic myotrophic and antigonadotrophic properties of some anabolic steroids, *Steroids,* 15, 61, 1970.
5. **Basulko, A. S.,** The Use of Nerabol by Intensive Muscular Activity of Strength (Statical) Character in the Experiments on Animals, Diss., Tartu Univ., 1974.
6. **Mainwaring, W. I. P.,** *The Mechanism of Action of Androgens,* Springer-Verlag, New York, 1977.
7. **Mainwaring, W. I. P., Wilce, P. H., and Smith, A. E.,** Studies on the form and synthesis of messenger ribonucleic acid in the rat ventral prostate gland, including its tissue-specific regulation by androgen, *Biochem. J.,* 137, 513, 1974.
8. **Ichil, S., Izawa, M., and Murakami, N.,** Hormonal regulation of protein synthesis in rat ventral prostate, *Endocrinology (Jap.),* 21, 267, 1974.
9. **Mainwaring, W. I. P. and Wilce, P. A.,** The control of the form and function of the ribosomes in androgen-dependent tissue by testosterone, *Biochem. J.,* 134, 795, 1973.
10. **Butler, W. W. S. and Schade, W. L.,** The effect of castration and androgenic replacement on the nucleic acid composition, metabolism and enzymatic capabilities of the rat ventral prostate, *Endocrinology,* 63, 271, 1958.
11. **Mainwaring, W. I. P., Mangan, F. R., Irving, R. A., and Jones, D. A.,** Specific changes in the messenger ribonucleic acid content of the rat ventral prostate gland after androgenic stimulation: evidence from the synthesis of aldolase messenger ribonucleic acid, *Biochem. J.,* 144, 413, 1974.
12. **Kochakian, C. D.,** Mechanism of androgen action, *Lab. Invest.,* 8, 538, 1959.
13. **Kochakian, C. D. and Endahl, B. R.,** Influence of androgens on transaminase activities of different tissues, *Am. J. Physiol.,* 186, 460, 1956.
14. **Kochakian, C. D.,** Regulation of muscle growth by androgens, in *The Physiology and Biochemistry of Muscle as a Food,* Brigsky, E. J., Cassens, R. G., and Trautman, J. C., Eds., The University of Wisconsin Press, Madison, 1966, 88.
15. **Sommerwille, J.,** RNA polymerase I promoters and transcription factors, *Nature,* 310, 189, 1984.
16. **Beelee, T. J. C. and Butterworth, P. H. W.,** Eukaryotic DNA-dependent RNA polymerases:

an evaluation of their role in the regulation of gene expression, in *Eukaryotic Gene Regulation*, Kolody, G. M., Ed., CRC Press, Boca Raton, FL, 1980, 179.

17. **Yu, F. and Fegelson, P.**, A rapid turnover of RNA polymerase of rat liver nucleolus and of its messenger RNA, *Proc. Natl. Acad. Sci. USA*, 69, 2833, 1972.

18. **Feldcoren, B. I. and Rogozkin, V. A.**, The effect of retabolil on DNA-dependent RNA-polymerase in skeletal muscles, in *Endocrine Mechanisms of Regulation of the Adaptation to Muscular Activities*, Tartu, 1977, 7.

19. **Rogozkin, V. A. and Feldcoren, B. I.**, The effect of retabolil and training on activity of RNA polymerase in skeletal muscle, *Med. Sci. Sports*, 11, 345, 1979.

20. **Feldcoren, B. I.**, The effect of retabolil and training on synthesis of ribosomal RNA in skeletal muscles, in *Medicine and Sports*, Research Institute of Physical Culture, Leningrad, 1979, 124.

21. **Scow, R. A. and Hagan, S. N.**, Effect of testosterone propionate on myosin, collagen and other protein fraction in striated muscles of gonadectomized male guinea pigs, *Am. J. Physiol.*, 180, 31, 1955.

22. **Basulko, A. S. and Rogozkin, V. A.**, The effect of nerabol on aspartate aminotransferase activity of rats skeletal muscles under the conditions of experimental training, *Ukr. Biochem. J.*, 45, 29, 1973.

23. **Chainey, G. B. N. and Kanugo, M. S.**, Effects of estradiol and testosterone in the activity of pyruvate kinase of the cardiac and skeletal muscles of rats as a function of age and sex, *Biochim. Biophys. Acta*, 540, 65, 1978.

24. **Koenig, H., Goldstone, A., and Lu, Ch.Y.**, Androgens regulate mitochondrial cytochrome C oxidase and lysosomal hydrolases in mouse skeletal muscle, *Biochem. J.*, 192, 349, 1980.

25. **Gepinath, R. and Kitts, N. D.**, Effect of anabolic compounds on plasma levels of nitrogenous compounds and hepatic levels of tyrosine aminotransferase in growing beef steers, *Am. Soc. Sci. West Sect.*, p. 225, 1981.

26. **Kontula, K. K., Torkkeli, T. K., Bardin, C. W., and Jänne, O. A.**, Androgen induction of ornithine decarboxylase mRNA in mouse kidney as studied by complimentary DNA, *Proc. Natl. Acad. Sci. USA*, 81, 731, 1984.

27. **Anderson, A. C., Hammer, L., Henningsson, S., and Lowendahl, G. O.**, Changes in cadaverine and putrescine metabolism in the mouse kidney induced to growth by an anabolic steroid, *Acta Physiol. Scand.*, 114, 225, 1982.

28. **Jänne, O., Isomaa, V., Pajunen, A., Wright, W., and Bardin, W.**, How changes in cytosol and nuclear androgen receptors relate to the testosterone responses: studies with new exchange assays, *Gene Reg. Steroid Hormones*, 2, 277, 1983.

29. **Yacovlev, N. N., Ed.**, *Biochemistry*, Text Book for Physical Culture Institutes, Phys. Cult. and Sports, Moscow, 1974.

30. **Goldberg, A. L., Etlinger, J. D., Goldspink, D. F., and Jablecki, C.**, Mechanism of work-induced hypertrophy of skeletal muscle, *Med. Sci. Sport*, 7, 248, 1975.

31. **Edington, D. N. and Edgerton, V. R.**, *The Biology of Physical Activity*, Houghton Mifflin, Boston, 1976.

32. **Stepanov, M. G.**, Androgens Reception by Isolated Nuclei of Skeletal Muscles and Its Change by Physical Exercises and 19-Nortestosterone Injection, Diss., Leningrad, 1984.

33. **Exner, G. U., Staude, H. W., and Pette, D.**, Isometric training of rats: effects upon fast and slow muscle and modifications by an anabolic hormone (nandrolone decanoate). I. Female rats, *Pfluger's Arch.*, 345, 1, 1973.

34. **Exner, G. U., Staude, H. W., and Pette, D.**, Isometric training of rats: effects upon fast and slow muscle and modification by an anabolic hormone (nandrolone decanoate). II. Male rats, *Pfluger's Arch.*, 345, 15, 1973.

35. **Stone, M. H. and Lipner, H.**, Responses to intensive training and methandrostenolone administration. I. Contractile and performance variables, *Pfluger's Arch.*, 375, 141, 1978.

36. **Stone, M. H., Rush, M. E., and Lipner, H.**, Responses to intensive training and methandro-stenolone administration. II. Hormonal, organ weights, muscle weight and body composition, *Pfluger's Arch.*, 375, 147, 1978.

37. **Doine, A. I. and Fava de Morales, F.,** Biochemical modulation of the submandibular gland of castrated male mice treated with anabolic steroids, *J. Biol. Buccale,* 9, 401, 1981.

38. **Max, S. R. and Toop, J.,** Androgens enhance in vivo 2-deoxyglucose uptake by rat striated muscle, *Endocrinology,* 113, 119, 1981.

39. **Samules, L. T., Matsumoto, K., and Samuels, B. K.,** Localization of enzymes involved in testosterone biosynthesis by the mouse testis, *Endocrinology,* 94, 55, 1974.

40. **Samules, L. T., Bussman, L., Matsumoto, K., and Huschby, R. A.,** Organization of androgen biosynthesis in the testis, *J. Steroid Biochem.,* 6, 291, 1975.

41. **Sato, B., Huseby, R. A., and Samules, L. T.,** The possible role of membrane organization in the activity of androgen biosynthesis enzymes associated with normal or tumorous Leydig cell microsomes, *Endocrinology,* 103, 805, 1978.

42. **Ewing, L. L., Zirkin, B. R., Cochran, R. C., Kromann, N., Peters, C., and Ruiz-Bravo, N.,** Testosterone secretion by rat, rabbit, guinea pig, dog and hamster testis perfused in vitro: correlation with Leydig cell mass, *Endocrinology,* 105, 1135, 1979.

43. **Zirkin, B. R., Ewing, L. L., Kromann, N., and Cochran, R. C.,** Testosterone secretion by rat, rabbit, guinea pig, dog and hamster testis perfused in vitro: correlation with Leydig cell ultrastructure, *Endocrinology,* 107, 1867, 1980.

44. **De Kretse, D. M.,** Changes in the fine structure of the human testicular interstitial cells after treatment with human gonadotrophins, *Z. Zellforsch. Mikrosk. Anat.,* 83, 344, 1967.

45. **Saartok, T., Dahlberg, F., and Gustafsson, J.-Å.,** Relative binding affinity of anabolic-androgenic steroids: comparison of the binding to the androgen receptors in skeletal muscle and in prostate, as well as to sex hormone-binding globulin, *Endocrinology,* 114, 2100, 1984.

46. **Bollard, F. J. and Geoffrey, L. F.,** Effects of anabolic agents on protein breakdown in L6 myoblasts, *Biochem. J.,* 210, 243, 1983.

47. **Buffery, P. J and Vernon, B. G.,** Protein metabolism in animals treated with anabolic agents, *Vet. Res. Commun.,* 7, 11, 1983.

48. **Harkonen, P.,** Androgenic control of glycolysis, the pentose cycle and pyruvate dehydrogenase in the rat ventral prostate, *J. Steroid Biochem.,* 14, 1075, 1981.

49. **Singhal, R. L., Parvleker, M. R., Vijayvarigiya, R., and Robinson G. A.,** Metabolic control mechanism in mammalian systems, *Biochem. J.,* 125, 329, 1971.

50. **Mangan, F. R., Pegg, A. E., and Mainwaring, W. I. P.,** A reappraisal of the effects of adenosine 3':5'-cyclic monophosphate on the function and morphology of the rat prostate gland, *Biochem. J.,* 134, 129, 1973.

51. **Rogozkin, V. A.,** Metabolic effect of anabolic steroid on skeletal muscle, *Med. Sci. Sports,* 11, 160, 1979.

52. **Rogozkin, V. A.,** Anabolic steroid metabolism in skeletal muscle, *J. Steroid Biochem.,* 11, 923, 1979.

53. **Litvinova, V. N. and Rogozkin, V. A.,** Reactions of organism of white rats of different age to influence of androgenic anabolic steroids, *Acta Comm. Univ. Tartuensis (USSR),* 562, 102., 1981.

54. **Rogozkin, V. A. and Feldcoren, B. I.,** Androgens and adaptation of the organism to physical exercises, in *Muscular Activity and Hormones,* Research Institute of Physical Culture, Leningrad, 1982, 6.

55. **Cato, A. C. B.,** How steroid hormones function to induce the transcription of specific genes, *Bio. Rep.,* 3, 101, 1983.

56. **King, W. J. and Greene, G. L.,** Monoclonal antibodies localize oestrogen receptor in the nuclei of target cells, *Nature,* 307, 745, 1984.

57. **Welshons, W. V., Lieberman, M. E., and Gorski, J.,** Nuclear localization of unoccupied oestrogen receptor, *Nature,* 307, 747, 1984.

58. **Payvar, F., Wrange, O., Carlstendt-Duke, J., Okret, S., Gustafsson, J.-O., and Yamomoto, K. R.,** Purified glucocorticoid receptors bind selectively in vitro to a cloned DNA fragment whose transcription is regulated by glucocorticoids in vivo, *Proc. Natl. Acad. Sci. USA,* 78, 6628, 1981.

59. **Campton, J. C., Schrader, W. T., and O'Malley, B. W.,** DNA sequence preference of the progesterone receptor, *Proc. Natl. Acad. Sci. USA,* 89, 16, 1983.
60. **Darnell, J. E.,** Variety in the level of gene control in eukaryotic cell, *Nature,* 297, 365, 1982.
61. **Gazarjan, K. G. and Tarantul, V. Z.,** *Eukaryotic Genome, Molecular Organization and Expression,* Moscow State University, Moscow, 1983.

Chapter 6

ENZYMIC SYSTEMS PARTICIPATING IN
AAS METABOLISM

The processes of AAS intracellular transformation are closely associated with androgen metabolism and the same enzymic systems take part in them. AAS are involved with hydrophobic substances and in the process of catabolic reactions they not only change their hormonal activity, but in this case the steroid molecules become more hydrophilic. By converting AAS molecules to a water-soluble substance, the majority of steroids are subjected to conjugation with sulphates or glucuronic acid and, in the form of conjugates, they are excreted from the organism. By examining the processes of AAS intracellular metabolism it should be taken into consideration that besides the hormones themselves, receptor proteins actively participate in them, too. The velocity of getting a hormone signal into a cell depends, in many respects, on the presence of these proteins and the processes which condition their interaction with AAS.

We considered it to be advisable to examine in this chapter the common enzymic systems participating in a biotransformation of both the AAS molecules and their receptors. One may distinguish four large classes of enzymes which take part in these processes in the organism. They are oxidoreductases, trans-ferases, hydrolases and isomerases. A few enzymes participating in AAS metabolism are given in Table 18 according to enzyme classification.[1]

Oxidoreductases

Oxidoreductases catalyze both direct and reversible reactions. They can reduce and oxidize substrates with the participation of reduced or oxidized nicotinamide-adenine dinucleotides (NADPH, NADP).

Within this large group of enzymes participating in AAS metabolism there are three subclasses with narrow specialization in the catalysis of certain types of reactions.[2-4] The first subclass of oxidoreductase enzymes acts on CH–OH steroid groups with the participation of NAD and NADP as acceptors. The second subclass of enzymes catalyzes direct dehydrogenation of CH–CH steroid groups and also involves NAD and NADP in the reactions. The third subclass are monooxidases which catalyze steroid oxidation with the participation of fla-voproteins and iron sulfur protein.

The first subclass of enzymes are the most common and are widely repre-sented in many tissues of an organism. The action of any enzyme of this group involves successive stages in which NAD or NADP is reduced by means of double-electronic transfer. This process involves taking the hydrate ion H⁻ from the oxidized steroid while the proton passes to the medium. Initially the binding of an enzyme to a co-enzyme (NAD or NADP) occurs. Then a triple complex is formed which includes the enzyme, the co-enzyme and a substrate (steroid). The

TABLE 18
Enzymes Involved in the Transformation of Steroids

Number	Recommended name	Reaction	Systematic name
1.	Oxidoreductase		
1.1.	Acting on CH–OH groups as donors		
1.1.1.	With NAD or NADP as acceptor		
1.1.1.50	3α-Hydroxysteroid dehydrogenase	Androsterone + NADP = 5α-androstane-3,17-dione + NADPH	3α-Hydroxysteroid: NADP oxidoreductase
1.1.1.51	β-Hydroxysteroid dehydrogenase	Testosterone + NADP = 4-androstene-3,17-dione + NADPH	3(or 17)β-Hydroxysteroid: NADP oxidoreductase
1.1.1.63	Testosterone 17β-dehydrogenase	Testosterone + NAD⁺ = 4-androstene-3,17-dione + NADH	17β-Hydroxysteroid: NAD 17-oxidoreductase
1.1.1.64	Testosterone 17β-dehydrogenase NADP	Testosterone + NADP⁺ = 4-androstene-3,17-dione + NADPH	17β-Hydroxysteroid: NADP 17-oxidoreductase
1.1.1.145	3β-Hydroxy-Δ⁵-steroid dehydrogenase	3β-Hydroxy-5-ene-steroid + NAD = 3-oxo-4-ene-steroid + NADH	3β-Hydroxy-5-ene-steroid: NAD + 3-oxidoreductase
1.1.1.146	11β-Hydroxysteroid dehydrogenase	11β-Hydroxysteroid + NADP = 11-oxosteroid + NADPH	11β-Hydroxysteroid: NADP 11-oxidoreductase
1.1.1.147	16α-Hydroxysteroid dehydrogenase	16α-Hydroxysteroid + NADP = 16-oxosteroid + NAD(P)H	16α-Hydrosteroid: NADP 16-oxidoreductase
1.1.1.152	Etiocholanolone 3α-dehydrogenase	Etiocholanolone + NAD = 5β-androstane-3,17-dione + NADH	3α-Hydroxy-5β-steroid: NAD 3-oxidoreductase
1.1.1.159	7α-Hydroxysteroid dehydrogenase	3α,7α,12α-Trihydroxy-5β-cholanate + NAD = 3α,12α-dihydroxy-7-oxo-5β-cholanate + NADH	7α-Hydroxy-5β-steroid: NAD 7α-oxidoreductase
1.1.1.176	12α-Hydroxysteroid dehydrogenase	3α,7α,12α-Trihydroxy-5β-cholanate + NADP = 3α,7α-dihydroxy-12-oxo-5β-cholanate + NADPH	12α-Hydroxysteroid: NAD 12α-oxidoreductase

1.3. Acting on CH–CH groups as donors

1.3.1. With NADP or NAD as acceptor

1.3.1.22	Cholesterone 5α-reductase	5α-Cholestan-3-one + NADP = cholest-4-en-3-one + NADPH	3-Oxo-5α-steroid: NADP 4-en-oxidoreductase
1.3.1.23	Cholesterone 5β-reductase	5β-Cholestan-3-one + NADP = cholest-4-en-3-one + NADPH	3-Oxo-5β-steroid: NADP 5β-oxidoreductase

1.3.99 With other acceptors

1.3.99.4	3-Oxosteroid Δ'-dehydrogenase	A 3-oxosteroid + acceptor = a 1-en-3-oxosteroid + reduced acceptor	3-Oxosteroid: (acceptor) 1-en-oxidoreductase
1.3.99.5	3-Oxo-5α-steroid Δ⁴-dehydrogenase	A 3-oxo-5α-steroid + acceptor = a 3-oxo-4-ene-steroid + reduced acceptor	3-Oxo-5α-steroid: (acceptor) 4-en-oxidoreductase
1.3.99.6	3-Oxo-5β-steroid Δ⁴-dehydrogenase	A 3-oxo-5β-steroid + acceptor = a 3-oxo-4-ene-steroid + reduced acceptor	3-Oxo-5β-steroid: (acceptor) 4-en-oxidoreductase

1.14 Acting on paired donors with incorporation of molecular oxygen

1.14.14 With reduced flavin or flavoprotein as one donor, and incorporation of one atom of oxygen

1.14.14.1	Flavoprotein-linked monooxygenase	RH + reduced flavoprotein + O_2 = ROH + oxidized flavoprotein + H_2O	RH, reduced-flavoprotein: oxygen oxidoreductase (RH-hydroxylating)

1.14.15 With a reduced iron-sulphur protein as one donor, and incorporation of one atom of oxygen

1.14.15.4	Steroid 11β-monooxygenase	A steroid + reduced adrenal ferredoxin + O_2 = an 11β-hydroxysteroid + oxidized adrenal ferredoxin + H_2O	Steroid, reduced ferredoxin: oxygen oxidoreductase (11β-hydroxylating)
1.14.15.5	Corticosterone 18-monooxygenase	Corticosterone + reduced adrenal ferrodoxin + O_2 = 18-hydroxycorticosterone + oxidized adrenal ferrodoxin + H_2O	Corticosterone, reduced ferredoxin: oxygen oxidoreductase (18-hydroxylating)

1.14.99 Miscellaneous (required further characterization)

1.14.99.4	Progesterone monooxygenase	Progesterone + AH_2 + O_2 = testosterone-acetate + A + H_2O	Progesterone, hydrogen-donor: oxygen oxidoreductase (hydroxylating)
1.14.99.9	Steroid 17α-monooxygenase	A steroid + AH_2 + O_2 = a 17α-hydroxysteroid + A + H_2O	Steroid, hydrogen-donor: oxygen oxidoreductase (17α-hydroxylating)

TABLE 18 (continued)
Enzymes Involved in the Transformation of Steroids

Number	Recommended name	Reaction	Systematic name
1.14.99.10	Steroid 21-hydroxylase	A steroid + AH_2 + O_2 = a 21-hydroxysteroid + A + H_2O	Steroid, hydrogen-donor: oxygen oxidoreductase (21-hydroxylating)
1.14.99.11	Estradiol 6β-monooxygenase	Estradiol-17β + AH_2 + O_2 = 6β-hydroxyestradiol + A + H_2O	Estradiol-17β, hydrogen donor: oxygen oxidoreductase (6β-hydroxylating)
1.14.99.12	4-Androstene-3,17-dione mono-oxygenase	Androst-4-ene-3,17-dione + AH_2 + O_2 = 13-hydroxy-3-oxo- + 3,17-secoandrost-4-en-17-oic (17→13)-lactone + A + H_2O	Androst-4-ene-3,17-dione, hydrogen donor: oxygen oxidoreductase (13-oxidoreductase, lactonizing)
1.14.99.14	Progesterone 11α-hydroxylase	Progesterone + AH_2 + O_2 = 11α-hydroxyprogesterone + A + H_2O	Progesterone, hydrogen-donor: oxygen oxidoreductase (11α-hydroxylating)
1.14.99.16	Methylsterol monooxygenase	4,4-Dimethyl-5-cholest-7-en-3-ol + AH_2 + O_2 = 4α-methyl-5α-cholest-7-en-3β-ol + A + H_2O	4,4-Dimethyl-5α-cholest-7-en-3β-ol, hydrogen-donor: oxygen oxidoreductase
2.	Transferases		
2.4.	Glycosyltransferases		
2.4.1	Hexosyltransferases		
2.4.1.59	UDP glucuronate-estradiol glucurono-syltransferase	UDP glucuronate + 17β-estradiol = UDP + 17β-estradiol 3d-glucuronoside	UDP glucuronate: 17β-estradiol 3-glucuronosyltransferase
2.4.1.61	UDP glucuronate-estradiol 16α-glucuronosyltransferase	UDP glucuronate + estradiol = UDP + estradiol 16α-mono-D-glucuronoside	UDP glucuronate: 16α-estradiol glucuronyltransferase
2.7.	Transferring phosphorus-containing groups		
2.7.1.	Phosphotransferase with alcohol group as acceptor		

EC number	Enzyme name	Reaction	Alternative name
2.7.1.37	Protein kinase	ATP + a protein = ADP + a phosphoprotein	ATP: protein phosphotransferase
2.7.7.	Nucleotidyltransferase		
2.7.7.4	Sulphate adenylyl transferase (ATP-sulphurylase)	ATP + sulphate = pyrophosphate + adenylylsulphate	ATP: sulphate adenylyltransferase
2.8	Transferring sulphur-containing groups		
2.8.2	Sulphotransferases		
2.8.2.2	3β-Hydroxysteroid sulphotransferase	3′-Phosphoadenylylsulphate + a 3β-hydroxysteroid = adenosine-3′,5′-biphosphate + a steroid-3β-sulphate	3′-Phosphoadenylylsulphate: 3β-hydroxysteroid sulphotransferase
3.	Hydrolases		
3.1.	Acting on ester bonds		
3.1.1.	Carboxylic ester hydrolases		
3.1.1.13	Cholesterol esterase	A cholesterol ester + H_2O = cholesterol + fatty acid anion	Sterol-ester acylhydrolase
3.1.3.	Phosphoric monoester hydrolase		
3.1.3.16	Phosphoprotein phosphatase	A phosphoprotein + n H_2O = a protein + n orthophosphate	Phosphoprotein phosphohydrolase
3.1.6.	Sulphuric ester hydrolases		
3.1.6.2	Sterol sulphatase	3β-Hydroxyandrost-5-en-17-one-3-sulphate + H_2O = 3β-hydroxyandrost-5-en-17-one + sulphate	Sterol-sulphate sulphohydrolase
3.2.	Glycosidases		
3.2.1.	Hydrolyzing O-glycosyl compounds		
3.2.1.31	β-D-Glucuronidase	A β-D-glucuronide + H_2O = an alcohol + D-glucuronate	β-D-Glucuronide glucuronosohydrolase
5.	Isomerases		
5.3.	Intermolecular oxidoreductase		
5.3.3.	Transposing C=C bonds		
5.3.3.1	Steroid Δ-isomerase	A 3-oxo-5-ene-steroid = a 3-oxo-4-ene-steroid	3-Oxosteroid 5 en-4-en-isomerase (3-oxosteroid Δ^5-Δ^4-isomerase)

dissociation of such a triple complex occurs in reverse order. First the steroid separates from the enzyme and thereupon the co-enzyme does the same. Each reduced NADH and NADPH contains one hydrogen carried from the steroid during the course of the reaction. The carrying over of hydrogen atoms by the enzymes is stereospecific with respect to the plane of a pyridine ring. The stereospecificity of hydrogen carrying over is defined by which side of this ring plane the steroid is bound to the enzyme. All the oxidoreductases catalyzing hydrogen transport from steroids to NAD and NADP pertain to β-type. The majority of enzymes manifest a catalytic activity with one co-enzyme. Because of this the velocity of the reaction considerably exceeds that of the reaction with another co-enzyme. One may talk about a specificity of enzymes to NAD or NADP.

In the microsomes of liver, kidneys, adrenals, testicles, and prostate, as well as in various bacteria forming a part of the intestinal flora, the enzymes accelerating hydroxylation reactions according to different positions of the steroid molecule are widely represented.[5–9] The hydroxylation reactions result in the formation of 2β-, 3-, 3α-, 6β-, 11β-, 16α-, and 17β-oxiderivatives of steroids.[10,11] Among the enzymes which participate in steroid transformation most intensively are 3α-hydroxysteroid dehydrogenase (EC 1.1.1.50), 3(17)β-hydroxysteroid dehydrogenase (EC 1.1.1.51) and 17β-hydroxysteroid dehydrogenase (EC 1.1.1.64). The first two enzymes were isolated from various tissues and purified by means of column chromatography.[12–14] It was shown that the enzymes differ in the degree of their interaction with the co-factors NADH and NADPH.[15,16] However, the presence of other similar physical-chemical properties shows that they may be identical proteins in at least sex organs (testicles, prostate, epididymis).[17] Both enzymes were also revealed in the cytoplasm of rat skeletal muscles.[18] Four isoenzymes of 3α-hydroxysteroid dehydrogenase (EC 1.1.1.50) with a molecular mass of 40,000 to 41,000 were obtained from the cytoplasm of rabbit kidneys and liver.[19,20] The isoenzymes have similar substrate specificity and characteristics. They are very similar in amino acid composition. This evidence allows us to consider them as the product of familial genes. 17β-Hydroxysteroid dehydrogenase also differs according to the degree of interaction with a co-factor in various tissues. In adrenals the enzyme uses NADH as a co-factor,[21] while in testicles it manifests a large affinity for NADPH while NADH proves to be inefficient.[22] The oxidation of the hydroxylic group in position 17 of AAS molecule to oxo group which occurs under the action of this enzyme leads to a rise in 17-oxo steroid concentration. Comparison of the values of 17-oxo steroid excretion with structural peculiarities of AAS molecule establishes that AAS, which were nonalkylated and which did not contain halogens, most actively participated in this reaction of oxidation.[23] The position of a double bond in ring A and the substitution of a methyl group in position 1, 2, and 6 of the steroid molecule proved to be a highly important fact. Essential differences in enzyme activity in various tissues may affect the velocity of diverse AAS metabolism. The highest enzyme activity was revealed in kidneys and liver,[24] while in prostate the enzyme practically does not interact with AAS. One may suppose the participation of other enzymes of this subclass in steroid biotransformation. However, necessary experimental evidence has not yet been obtained.

The second subclass includes the enzymes introducing a double bond into the steroid molecule by means of a direct dehydrogenation of a CH-CH bond. In this group of enzymes, particular attention was given to the study of 5α-reductase (EC 1.3.1.22) and 5β-reductase (EC 1.3.1.23). The first investigations showed that in the process of the reaction 5α-dihydrotestosterone was formed from testosterone under the action of the 5α-reductase enzyme.[25,26] A distinctive peculiarity of this reaction is an enzymatic introduction of a double bond into ring A of the steroid molecule which occurs only in the presence of $NADP^+$.[27] The enzyme is revealed in the microsomal fraction of liver, kidneys, adrenals, testicles and prostate.[4,28,29] A detailed study of enzyme localization in prostate revealed an irregularity of its distribution between various cells.[30] In epithelial cells, the activity of 5α-reductase and 3α-hydroxysteroid dehydrogenase proved to be considerably higher than in stromal cells.[31,32] It points out the differences in the velocity of testosterone metabolism in various tissues of glands and may be used during the evaluation of its functional state.[33] Some differences were seen in the substrate specificity of the enzyme localized in liver and prostate. The velocity of this reaction is limited by the concentration of free testosterone in the cell. Prostate 5α-dihydrotestosterone is an active androgen passing a hormonal signal inside the organ and for other target cells, such as skeletal muscle, testosterone and AAS serve as an active androgen. In skeletal muscle the activity of 5α-reductase is very low and a number of experiments do not reveal it at all. Four enzymes participating in androgen metabolism are revealed in human leukocytes: 5α-reductase and 3α-, 3β- and 17β-hydroxysteroid oxidoreductase.[34] The activity of these enzymes differs according to sex and age in a human being. 5β-Reductase is localized in the microsomal fraction of liver, adrenals, and testicles. The enzyme has a strict co-factor specificity and only $NADP^+$ participates in the reaction. The main function of this enzyme is also associated with testosterone metabolism and leads to the formation of 5β-androsterone (etiocholanolone), which is excreted from the organism.

Monooxygenases

In recent years there has been revealed, in various tissues, a system of enzymes that catalyze the transition of lipid-soluble substances, including AAS, into water-soluble combinations which are easily excreted from an organism. This group of enzymes catalyze the reduction of flavoproteins or iron sulfur proteins with the inclusion of molecular oxygen. A sufficiently high activity in the microsomal fraction of flavoprotein-bound monooxidase liver cells (EC 1.14.14.1) may be noted. The activity of another group of liver microsomal enzymes was determined by the interaction of its basic components, membrane-bound proteins of cytochrome P_{450} and NADPH-cytochrome P_{450}-reductase (EC 1.6.2.4).

By introducing various AAS into an organism, the reversible activity of the liver monooxidase system may increase. There exists a certain molar ratio of NADPH-cytochrome P_{450}-reductase to cytochrome P_{450} which may be altered. Monooxygenases are membrane-bound enzymes and their organization and function in biological membranes are defined by the conditions of localization. The molecule of NADPH-cytochrome P_{450}-reductase is supposed to be surrounded by several cytochrome P_{450} molecules in a biological membrane and represents a structural organization of the microsomal monooxygenase system.[35,36] In the first stage of the reaction, AAS binds to cytochrome P_{450} (Fe^{3+}) which was oxidized from the formation of the cytochrome P_{450}-steroid complex (Figure 20). Later on there occurs the reduction of cytochrome P_{450} due to the electron passed by NADPH which catalyzes flavoprotein-cytochrome P_{450}-reductase. The enzyme has a molecular mass of 78,000 and it is localized in the membrane. In the composition of the enzyme there is one molecule of FAD and one of FMN. The reduced form of cytochrome P_{450} produces an oxidized intermediate product. Then, by passing the electron from cytochrome b_5, reduction takes place and interacts with the oxidized intermediate product. It results in the formation of a hydroxylic steroid that is an oxidized form of cytochrome P_{450} and water. Under the action of monooxygenase system an intensive formation of hydroxylic steroids occurs and they enter the reaction of conjugation and are excreted from the organism. Multiple forms of cytochrome P_{450} are revealed in liver microsomes. They have marked structural differences, a diverse molecular mass, and various absorption spectra in ultraviolet and visible light.[36,37] The isoenzymes of cytochrome P_{450} also possess various affinities for specific substrates and a diverse ability to interact with cytochrome b_5.[38] In liver, a group of enzymes, with the participation of cytochrome P_{450}, pertain to induced proteins and their number may be altered within large limits by the introduction of various substances, including medicines and steroids, into the organism. There exists some evidence

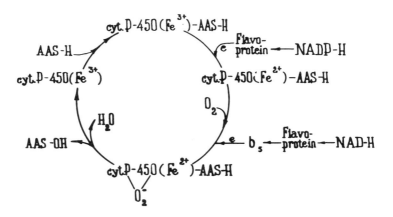

FIGURE 20.   AAS hydroxylation in the system of cytochrome P-450.

for the presence of selective induction of cytochrome P_{450} of separate forms in humans.[39] In the cortex of adrenals, the cytochrome P_{450} is localized in the membrane of mitochondria and catalyzes the reaction of AAS hydroxylation in position 11β. It should be noted that in this tissue, the electrons are transported to cytochrome P_{450} not from flavoprotein but from adrenodoxine iron sulfur protein. The reduction of adrenodoxine occurs with the participation of the NADPH-dependent adrenodoxine reductase enzyme and within its structure there is a molecule of FAD.

The system of monooxygenases, which is situated in sex organ microsomal membranes, catalyzes the synthesis of androgens from progesterone with the participation of cytochromes P_{450}.[40,41] Under the action of steroid 17α-monooxygenase enzyme (EC 1.14.99.4) the conversion of progesterone to 17α-hydroxyprogestone occurs. The enzyme 17,20-lyase (EC 4.1) then catalyzes the rupture of the bond between positions 17 and 20 of the steroid molecule. Both reactions take place in the presence of cytochrome P_{450}.[42,43] Cytochrome b_5 participates in the reaction as a donor of electrons.[44] The third enzymic system, the aromatase one, catalyzes the conversion of androgens to estrogens.[45] The enzymic mechanism of estrogen formation includes two successive hydroxylations of the C_{10} methyl group and hydroxylation in the C_2 position. It leads to the loss of a C_{10} methyl group in the form of formic acid with the elimination of hydrogens 1β and 2β (1β and 2β hydrogens) and the aromatization of steroid molecule ring A.[46,47] The hydroxylation occurs with the participation of three oxygen molecules and NADPH under the action of cytochrome P_{450} and NADPH-cytochrome P_{450}-reductase.[48] To discover the kinetic parameters of this multistage reaction, specific inhibitors interacting with steroid molecule C_{10} group were used.[49] By using testosterone with ^{18}O in position 3, over 90% of ^{18}O was recovered in the final product, estradiol.[50] Not only NADPH, but also NADH, can participate as co-factors in this reaction. However, in the latter case, the velocity of the reaction is considerably slower.[51] The aromatization of steroids into estrogens is closely associated with the state of the energy-dependent processes in mitochondria which maintain ATP intracellular funds.[52] The results of studies of AAS metabolism show that, in sex organs, the monooxygenase system of enzymes bound to cytochrome P_{450} catalyze the reactions of steroid hydroxylation in positions 6α, 7α, and 6β.[53] The regulation of androgen synthesis in sex organs is not only under the control of hypophyseal hormone but also depends on the state of the monooxidase systems. Testosterone can regulate the reaction of hydroxylation catalyzed by microsomal enzymes and cause alterations in cytochromes P_{450}.[54]

Isomerases

The enzymes of this group catalyze the intracellular migrations of C=C bond in a steroid molecule. Steroid isomerase (EC 5.3.3.1), which carries out the migration of the double bond from position 4.5 to position 5.6, has been studied the most. The enzyme is localized in the microsomal fraction of liver, adrenals, testicles, and placenta, as well as in a number of microorganisms. Some isomerases catalyzing the intramolecular migrations in the molecules of 5-androstenedione, 5-pregnene-3,20-dione and 17-hydroxy-5-pregnene-3,20-dione were demonstrated. The mechanism of action of these enzymes was studied in sufficient detail.[55] The reaction of a double bond migration consists of three stages and includes the proton transportation from position 4β to position 6β. These enzymes do not require the participation of co-factors; however they are inhibited by progesterone and estradiol.

Enzymic Systems of AAS Conjugation

All steroid hormones including AAS are excreted in an organism mainly in the form of conjugates with sulfuric and glucuronic acids. In a free form the steroids and their metabolites in urine make up 1%, with approximately 20 to 40% excreted in the conjugate form as glucuronic acid and more than 40% in the form of steroid sulphates.

Sulphotransferases

This group of enzymes catalyze the conversions of certain steroids to corresponding sulphates. They are found in many types of mammalian cells.[56,57] Two enzymes, sulphate-adenylyl-transferase (EC 2.7.7.4) and 3β-hydroxysteroid-sulphotransferase (EC 2.8.2.2), that participate in the biosynthesis of steroid sulphates have been purified and studied in detail. The enzymes are localized chiefly in the cells of liver and testicles. In these tissues a considerable part of the enzymes are bound to the endoplasmic reticulum and may be released after processing with detergents.[58,59] The study of substrate specificity established that among all the polyhydroxylic steroids, the reaction of sulfurization is carried out most intensively with 3-hydroxysteroids. Within this group of substances, 3β-steroids interact with the enzyme better than their 3α-forms.[60] Dihydroepiandrosterone proved to be the most specific substrate, and its use revealed several forms of enzymes differeing in their interaction with substrates.[61] It turned out that a sulphotransferase steroid differed from phenosulphotransferases.[62] Additionally, some differences with respect to such substrates as dihydroepiandrosterone and estrone were demonstrated inside this group of enzymes.[63,64] The reaction of steroid sulfurization proceeds at pH 7.7 and requires the presence of Mg ions. The sulphokinase reaction includes a successive proceeding of at least three stages with the participation of various enzymes and substrates. In the first stage, the enzyme ATP-sulfurylase (EC 2.7.7.4) catalyzes the formation of adenylylsulphate (adenosine-5-phosphosulphate, APS) which occurs in the presence of ATP. Then the phosphorylation of adenosine-5-phosphosulphate occurs with the same enzyme adenylyl-sulphate kinase and, in the presence of ATP, forms phosphoadenosine-5-phosphosulphate (PAPS). In the final stage, 3β-hydroxysteroid-sulphotransferase (EC 2.8.2.2) catalyzes the transfer of activated sulphate to the steroid hydroxylic group:

$$ATP + SO_4^{2-} \rightleftharpoons APS + PP \tag{5}$$
$$\text{ATP - sulfurylase}$$

$$APS + ATP \rightleftharpoons PAPS + ADP \tag{6}$$
$$\text{APS - kinase}$$

$$PAPS + R - OH \longrightarrow R - O - SO_3^- + PAP + H^+ \tag{7}$$
$$\text{hydroxysteroid - sulfotransferase}$$

Data on the kinetics of the reaction of steroid sulfurization in liver and testicles show that by retaining the total physical-chemical parameters (reaction velocity, pH, temperature) there were some differences due to the metabolic specific character of the tissue. Steroid sulfurization in liver is necessary for steroid detoxification and the subsequent excretion of hormones and their metabolites from the organism. The accumulation of steroid sulphates may lead to disturbance of the hormonal balance and thus they are rapidly removed from liver, no longer participating in metabolism. The biosynthesis of steroid sulphates in testicles and adrenals is tightly associated with the synthesis of androgens and 16-androstene derivatives, which is why the activity of 3β-hydroxysteroid-sulphotransferase is highest here.[65]

A noncompetitive inhibition of sulphotransferase activity in testicle and adrenal microsomes by the final product of the reaction (steroid sulphates) may be considered as a possible regulatory mechanism that controls the biosynthesis of androgens by means of the formation of 3β-hydroxysteroids and their sulphate ethers.[66,67]

Glucuronyltransferases

These enzymes catalyze the conversion of steroids to corresponding glucuronides. In mammals, such enzymes are found in a soluble fraction of many cells.[68,69] Two enzymes participating in the biosynthesis of steroid glucuronides were isolated from various tissues and studied. These are UDP-glucuronate-estradiol glucuronosyltransferase (EC 2.4.1.59) and UDP-glucuronate-estradiol 16α-glucuronosyltransferase (EC 2.4.1.61). The enzymes are localized in the membranes of liver cell endoplasmic reticulum. The reaction proceeds by means of the transfer of a glucuronide radical from uridine diphosphoglucuronic acid (UDPGA) to a steroid as follows:

$$UDPGA + \text{steroid} - OH \rightarrow \text{steroid-glucuronide} + UDP$$
$$\text{glucuronosyltransferase}$$

Recently, glucuronosyltransferase has been isolated from liver cells in a homogenous form and its molecular weight has been determined to be 57,000 daltons.[70]

On the basis of the study of enzyme substrate specificity a hypothesis was formed as to the presence of two forms of the enzyme that differ in their interaction with different groups of steroids. It was shown that in fact one of the glucuronyltransferase forms preferentially interacted with estrogens while the other form catalyzes androgen conversions.[71,72] These two enzymes were separated on columns with DEAE-cellulose and KM-cellulose.[73] The enzyme which catalyzes androgen conversion did not interact with estrene and estradiol. It was established that the activity of steroid transferases (both androgenic and estregenic) depends on the presence of phospholipids, and the removal of lipids during the purification of enzymes leads to a loss in their activity. Thus, glucuronyltransferases pertain to phospholipid-dependent enzymes and their activity is closely associated with the presence of phospholipids, in particular phosphatidylcholine.[74,75] Glucuronosyltransferase, catalyzing the conversion of estrogens, is regulated by the content of substrates and pertains to inducing enzymes. By introducing estradiol-17β into an organism, the activity of enzyme in liver essentially increases. The enzymes catalyzing the conversion of androgens are conservative enzymes, and hence their activity does not change after castration or testosterone injection.[74] Aside from enzyme participation in the synthesis of steroid conjugates, there exists a group of enzymes in various organic tissues which allow the hydrolysis of steroid conjugates.

Sulphatases

This group of enzymes catalyzes the hydrolysis of steroid hormone sulphates. The enzymes are found in the microsomal fraction of liver, adrenals, and sex glands.[56] In liver, sterol sulphatase possesses the highest activity (EC 3.1.6.2) and mainly hydrolyzes 3β-hydroxysteroid sulphate ethers. It was established that the activity of the liver microsomal enzyme is regulated by the level of androgens in the organism.[76] The change in excretion velocity of testosterone by endrogenic glands is reflected by sterol sulphatase activity in the liver.

Glucuronidase

The enzyme EC 3.2.1.31 catalyzes glucuronidase hydrolysis of various steroids. The largest amounts of enzyme are found in the cells of intestinal mucus membrane.[77] Study of enzyme substrate specificity showed that the velocity of steroid conjugate hydrolysis depended on the structure of the steroid and the junction of glucuronic acid. The velocity of steroid conjugate hydrolysis is gradually reduced by the presence of glucuronic acid in position C_3: $C_{3\beta} > C_{17\beta} > C_{3\alpha}$.[78] If it is necessary to carry out the hydrolysis of all conjugated AAS, located in blood or urine, an extract of mollusk juice *(Helix pomatia)* is usually used, which contains high sulfatase and glucuronidase activity.

The basic modification of steroid hormone receptors is associated with the processes of their phosphorylation. Therefore it is advisable to examine some groups of enzymes that participate in these reactions.

The phosphorylation of steroid receptors catalyzes the enzymes of protein kinase (EC 2.7.1.37). In mammalian tissues, several types of protein kinases have been found. They differ in molecular weight, subunit structure, substrate specificity and the character of their interaction with various activators. The classification of protein kinases is based on the ability of different effectors to alter the activity of these enzymes.[79,80] At present, the following protein kinases are known: cyclic AMP-dependent protein kinase types I and II, cyclic GMP-dependent protein kinases, Ca^{2+}-dependent protein kinases (Ca^{2+}-calmodulin-dependent and Ca^{2+}-diacetylglyceride-dependent), protein kinases which are dependent on two-chain RNA and nonspecific or independent protein kinases. Among this large group of enzymes, Ca^{2+}-calmodulin-dependent protein kinase is the one that phosphorylates steroid receptors. This enzyme has a sufficiently wide specificity taking part in the phosphorylation of microtube and neurofilament proteins, light myosin chains, smooth, heart, and skeletal muscle, and the proteins of synthetic membranes and those of steroid hormones receptors.[81–83] The enzyme activity depends on the presence of two effectors, calmodulin and Ca^{2+} ions. Calmodulin represents an acidic, heat-resistant protein with mw = 18,000.[84] The physical-chemical properties and the amino acid composition of calmodulin isolated from various sources are practically the same. The study of the reaction mechanism showed that it proceeds in two stages. In the first stage, through an interaction of the calmodulin molecule with four Ca ions, an intermediate complex is formed which interacts with the enzyme and activates it. The presence of Ca^{2+}-calmodulin-dependent protein kinase in various tissues opens the possibilities for phosphorylating various proteins including steroid hormone receptors.

Phosphoprotein Phosphatases

This group of enzymes (EC 3.1.3.16) catalyzes the dephosphorylation of various proteins including steroid hormone receptors.

Phosphoprotein phosphatases (PhPases) have been found in many mammalian tissues, among them liver, kidneys, adrenals, spleen, erythrocytes, heart and skeletal muscles.[85–87] PhPase localization is not limited to inside the cell; on the contrary, these enzymes have been found in a variety of cellular structures including cytoplasm,[87] mitochondria,[88] nucleus, nucleolus[89] and chromatin.[90] The substrate specificity of PhPases is very wide and includes a considerable number of proteins of different functional purposes and various molecular weights and phosphate groups. The velocity of phosphoprotein dephosphorylation may be determined by the nature of phosphorylated amino acid as well as its location in the protein molecule. PhPases can intensively catalyze the hydrolysis of a phosphate group from serine, threonine and tyrosine.[91,92] The presence of multiple forms and a molecular mass ranging from 12,000 to 500,000 may be considered as a distinctive peculiarity of these enzymes.[93] Most PhPase high molecular forms are formed by the association of a catalytic subunit, with various regulator proteins which alter substrate specificity and enzyme activity.[94] The catalytic PhPase subunit was isolated and purified from many tissues, and in most cases its molecular mass makes up about 35,000.[93] A high molecular form of PhPase, derived from pig heart, consists of three subunits α, β and γ with mw of 31,000, 80,000 and 62,000, respectively.[95] Only subunit α possesses a catalytic activity, while subunits β and γ are regulator proteins.

The presence of PhPase in various cell nuclei is of great significance for hormone steroid metabolism. It has been established that enzymes localized in cellular nuclei possess wide substrate specificity and catalyze the dephosphorylation of numerous acidic and basic phosphorylated proteins.[96] The activity of nuclear PhPases is regulated by a number of low molecular substances and metal ions. Among them are substances containing SH groups, molybdate, fluoride and others.

Among the proteins that are subjected to dephosphorylation by nuclear PhPases, steroid hormone receptors should be included. A number of investigations have shown that the dephosphorylation of estrogen receptors in the nucleus leads to the disintegration of the hormone-receptor complex.[97–99] Our experiments have also shown the possibility of a nuclear PhPase participating in the process of androgen-receptor complex inactivation in skeletal muscles which is accompanied by the reduction of androgen-binding activity. Thus, PhPases can participate in the process of receptor protein dephosphorylation and control the content of receptors in the cell. The participation of PhPases and protein kinases in steroid-hormone receptor phosphorylation and dephosphorylation not only confirms the conception of the receptor cycle in a cell but also changes it from an autonomous process to an energy-dependent process associated with many reactions of intracellular metabolism and with the reactions, accumulation and use of ATP funds.

Although findings on the study of AAS metabolism do not give a complete picture of each steroid transformation in an organism, they nevertheless demonstrate distinctive features of some AAS groups. The metabolism of 19-nortestosterone, for example, and its basic derivatives occurs with the participation of the same enzymic systems that catalyze testosterone degradation. The presence of an alkyl group in position 17α, a methyl group in position 1, and chlorine in position 4 in the structure of AAS molecules, as well as the presence of an additional double bond in ring A by C_1, retards the velocity of 17β-hydroxy group oxidation and affects the intensity of such steroid metabolism. The outlined method of AAS metabolism should be considered only a potential possibility; it does not mean that the metabolism of other AAS will occur similarly. The principal peculiarity of the metabolism of androgens, and their synthetic analogues — AAS, is in close connection with the intracellular metabolism of concrete tissues or organs. The clearly expressed dependence on characteristic features associated with the function of a target cell leads to essential differences in metabolic conversions of the same steroid in various tissues.

The classification of AAS shown in Chapter 1 demonstrates not only the peculiarities of the chemical structure of AAS, placing it in one of several groups, but also develops some potential metabolic pathways. Comparison of the structure of separate AAS inside the series and the groups shows that as a rule the differences between them consist of location and the number of separate chemical radicals. It leads us to believe, with great probability, that the metabolism processes of such AAS groups have great similarities. Some possible differences in the biotransformation of these hormones occur in the first stages. They are associated with the modification of separate functional groups. The truth of such a conclusion may be shown by the example of 19-nortestosterone derivative subgroups in which 14 steroids were obtained by means of 14 various chemical radicals by introduction of a 17β-OH group. It has been established that all of the derivatives of 19-nortestosterone have similar final metabolites. After injecting various derivatives of 19-nortestosterone only 19-norandrosterone and 19-noretiocholanolone are seen in urine.

The results of the study of AAS metabolism confirm the variety of initial reactions of their biotransformation in an organism and additionally show that the synthesis of many new AAS is carried out without a thorough investigation of possible steroid transformations. Some metabolites seen in the organism, in the process of AAS biotransformation, are given in Table 19.

As Table 19 shows, from a large AAS group of androstenic series, the metabolites of only three steroids are seen. From the androstane series, four steroids were studied and the derivatives of the estrene series have been the most thoroughly investigated. In the specimen of estrene series not only the community of chemical structures, but also that of metabolism were shown. In the specimen of the first group the same metabolites of norethandrolone and ethylestrenol were also revealed.[107] It has been established that according to its chemical structure, ethylestrenol differs from norestrandrolone only in the absence of oxygen in position C_3 of ring A. In an organism, after oxidation ethylestrenol turns into norethandrolone and the subsequent metabolism proceeds like the steroid.

The variety of metabolic pathways may be explained by this concept according to which any change in the chemical structure of a steroid hormone may be due to an unequal influence of cellular enzymes on the metabolism of the steroid molecules.[109] This thesis is confirmed by the investigation of the effect of natural steroids and their synthetic derivatives on the isomerization of 5-androstane-3,17-dione under the action of steroid-Δ-isomerase (EC 5.3.3.1).[110] It has been established that the presence of any substituent of C_{18}, C_{19} and C_{21} steroids in position C_{11} ("α" or "β") prevents their interaction with the enzyme. The presence of methyl, hydroxyl, ethyl and aceto groups in position C_{17} appreciably decreases the affinity of the steroid for the enzyme. In the case of C_{18}-C_{19} steroids, the absence of a methyl group in position C_{19}, as well as the presence of double bonds in positions C_9 or C_9 and C_{11}, lead to better binding to the enzyme. The metabolites of methandienone 17-epimethandrostenolone and 6β-hydroxymethylandrostenolone have been isolated and identified from human urine.[104,105]

TABLE 19
Metabolites of Some AAS

Series	Steroids	Metabolites	Ref.
Androstane	Drostanolone	2α-; 15α-; 16-Drostanolone	100
	Metenolone	3α-Hydroxymetenolone	101
	Oxandrolone	no	102
	Stanozolol	no	102
Androstene	Methandienone	6β-Hydroxymethandienone	103—105
	Chlostebol	3α-Hydroxychlostebol	105
	Turinabol	6β-Hydroxyturinabol	106
		6β,12-Dihydroxyturinabol	
		6β,16-Dihydroxyturinabol	
Estrene	19-Nortestosterone (nandrolone)	19-Norandrosterone	107
		19-Noretiocholanolone	
		19-Nortestosterone	
	Nandrolone-decanoate	19-Nortestosterone	107
	Nandrolone-phenylpropionate	19-Norandrosterone	107
		19-Noretiocholanolone	
	Norethandrolone	3α,5α-Tetraoxynorethandrolone, 3α,5β-tetraoxynorethandrolone, oxytetrahydronorethandrolone, oxynorethandrolone	107
	Ethylestrenol	Norethandrolone 17α-ethyl-5-estrane-3ξ,17β-diol	108

The biological effect on an organism is supposed to be manifested by not only methandienone itself but also by its active metabolites. According to its activity, the metabolite of methandienone 17β-hydroxy-17α-methyl-Δ'-androsten-3-one exerts a stronger action than does AAS.[103] An analogous action may also be seen for the other metabolite of methandienone, 3β,17β-dihydroxy-17α-methyl-Δ'-androstene. The biological effect is determined by the stability of ring A in the structure of the substance.[107] It has been established that reduction of the Δ⁴ bond in Δ¹,⁴-3-keto steroids precedes that of Δ' but not conversely. A high formation of metabolites with α,β-unsaturated 3-keto group from methandienone just due to Δ'-3-keto derivatives may apparently confirm this.[103]

The other specimen of the group of testosterone derivatives is methylandrostendiol. Study of metabolism in the tissue of rat adrenals showed that 17α-methyltestosterone, as well as 11-oxy-17α-methyltestosterone and hydroxylated derivatives of 17α-methyltestosterone, may be the basic product of steroid conversion. 17α-Methyl-5α-androstane-3α,17β-diol, 17α-methyl-5α-androstane-3β,17β-diol, 17α-methyl-5β-androstane-3α,16α,17β-triol, 17α-methyl-5β-androstane-3α,16β,17β-triol and the new metabolite 17α-methyl-5α-androstane-3α,6α,17β-triol were found in urine after injection of 17α-methyltestosterone into the organism.[111]

Injection of another AAS, such as drostanolone, into rabbits causes not only the reduction and the oxidation of oxygen-containing functional groups of 3 and 17 carbon atom, but also hydroxylation in positions 16α, 15α, and 2α of steroid structure.[100] The metabolites of such AAS as norethandrolone and ethylestrenol from the group of 19-nortestosterone derivatives have been studied in detail. After taking norethandrolone, it made up 36% of identified metabolites in human urine, while 16% was 3α,5α-tetraoxynorethandrolone, 15% was 3α,5β-tetraoxynorethandrolone, 20% was oxynorethandrolone, and 12% was oxytetrahydronorethandrolone.[107]

It was shown that ethylestrenol gives the same hydroxylated metabolites as norethandrolone itself. The presence of norethandrolone and ethylestrenol metabolites with a hydroxylic group in positions 6 and 7 (ring B) was proposed.[102]

The synthetic steroid linestrenol is also similar to ethylestrenol based on its structure and one may note that initally they are oxidized up to 3-oxi-4-en steroids.[103] By studying the metabolism of these AAS, an intensive hydroxylation of the ethylestrenol and norethandrolone side chain was demonstrated. The substances containing an ethylic group in the side chain metabolize, leaving the steroid hydroxylated in positions 1β, 2α, 6α, 10β, 16α, and 16β.[107] 19-Noretiocholanolone and 19-nortestosterone may be the basic metabolites of nandrolonedecanoate.

By studying AAS metabolism in an organism, the processes of steroid hormone intertransformations may be of certain significance. At present there are two principal pathways of metabolic transformation which have been the most intensively investigated. The first pathway is associated with the possibility of basic active metabolite transformations of adrenal cortex-androstenediol into testosterone. The increase in concentration of testosterone and its active metabolite, 5α-dihydrotestosterone, may result from not only the synthesis of these hormones in androgen-dependent tissues but also from metabolic transformations from androstenediol. The second pathway is associated with possible metabolic transformations of androgens to estrogens, which is of essential importance in the mechanism of androgen action as well. The enzymic system which causes the aromatization of androgens into estrogens is represented widely enough in various human and animal tissues. The possibility of the conversion of not only testosterone but also a number of AAS such as 19-nortestosterone and its derivative methandienone and others into estrogens was shown. Other AAS, such as metenolone and other steroids having a 17-hydroxy group, do not have to be subjected to the aromatization into estrogens. It was also shown that androstenediol is aromatized considerably more intensively into estrogen in human skeletal muscle than testosterone. The biological significance of androgen conversion into estrogens is highly significant and may exert an influence on different enzymic systems.

It has been established that the conversion of testosterone into estradiol in skeletal muscle is possible. Ultimately it causes a considerable increase in glucose-6-phosphate dehydrogenase activity.[111] The investigation of this reaction showed that fluoxymesterone, which was not subjected to aromatization, did not influence enzyme activity. The increase of glucose-6-phosphate dehydrogenase can occur by a direct 17β-estradiol injection and is inhibited by estrogens and not by androgen antagonists. The effect of testosterone on the activity of glucose-6-phosphate dehydrogenase may be blocked during the inhibition of the enzymes of aromatase systems.

While examining the facts determining the fate of AAS in an organism, steroid adsorption, which is closely associated with the place and method of hormone introduction, should be taken into account. There also is the factor of steroid distribution in various tissues, which is highly variable and tightly associated with the intracellular metabolism of a target cell. The transformation of steroids into active and inactive metabolites is completed by the liver and removal of these substances from the organism through the kidneys. Aside from the specific action due to the molecular structure, AAS may affect the state of metabolism in an organism by means of a change in the concentration of other endogenic, anabolic, and catabolic hormones, such as growth hormone, insulin, thyroxine, and corticosteroids. It has also been established that AAS may take a direct part in oxidation-reduction enzymic reactions. The ability of liver enzymes to catalyze AAS transformation is chiefly determined by the molecular structure of these hormones. It is the author's opinion that AAS function in an organism is widely represented in intracellular metabolism of various organs and tissues. AAS influence the growth of many tissues in organisms but by varying degrees. The action of AAS is carried out through an enzymic apparatus of the target cell. AAS easily penetrate the target cells, primarily sex organs and skeletal muscles, and after interaction with receptors they form hormone-receptor complexes which are transported to the nucleus and cause the expression of diverse genes. When all the receptors are saturated with hormones, any subsequent increase in AAS concentration will not result in an intensification of the hormonal signal effect. Such a situation may be considered to be a threshold of cellular concentration or an optimum for AAS which causes a maximum (highest possible) cellular effect. As long as this optimal concentration of intracellular AAS is unknown, one may believe that it is closely associated with the presence of androgen receptors and to some extent proportional to the steroid concentration in blood. As stated above, the concentration of AAS in tissues is closely related to the form of the steroid introduced. Peroral or parenteral AAS introduction into an organism is usually used. The investigation of AAS anabolic action has divided all these steroids into oral and injective ones,[23] although such a division appears to be relative.[112] Table 20 represents basic AAS used by various means of introduction into an organism.

A free AAS form has some advantages since it allows the regular maintenance of the necessary concentration of hormone in blood. However this form of AAS is rapidly subjected to metabolism in the stomach, and through the portal vein it gets to the liver and is excreted from the organism. Calculations show that the

TABLE 20
Basic AAS Used in Clinical Medicine

Oral	Injective
Oxandrolone	Metenolone-acetate
Oxymetholone	Methyltestosterone
Methandienone	19-Nortestosterone-phenylpropionate
Stanozolol	19-Nortestosterone
Testosterone-	19-Nortestosterone-propionate
decanoate	19-Nortestosterone-decanoate
Ethylestrenol	

half-life of testosterone in blood is only 4.7 min, trenbolone — 4 to 5 min, progesterone — 3.5 min and estradiol — 1.8 to 6.8 min.[114] This short half-life of a number of AAS leads to the necessity of carefully choosing the method of AAS introduction and dose during their use in clinical medicine and in cattle breeding. To raise the effectiveness of AAS action the mixture of several AAS or a mixture of AAS with natural sex hormones (testosterone, estradiol or progesterone) is used. The optimum regime of the use of AAS should ensure a maximum effect with a minimum risk of collateral action. This principle can be realized due to the most typical and common property of AAS, that of selective action. It is manifested by the fact that the sensitivity of some systems to hormones (sex systems, skeletal muscles) exceeds the sensitivity of other systems of vital importance. To create an optimum regime of AAS use in clinical medicine, a pharmacological model may be used.[115] In this case, control of the medical effect of AAS is carried out on the basis of the data of steroid concentration in the blood, which is more rapid and more reliable than determination of the final effect. The control for the final effect of AAS still needs more rapid methods of determination, a few of which are described in Chapters 8 and 9. The processes of steroid hormone biotransformation, including AAS, may be divided into two categories.[116] The first concerns the reactions where one functional group of steroid molecules is converted into another one or polar groups are introduced into the structure of nonpolar steroids. In this case the chemical nature of the corresponding reaction consists of oxidation or reduction, as well as hydrolysis. The second category of reactions is associated with the processes of the conjugation of steroid polar groups, mainly with sulphates and glucuronic acid. The reactions of the first group are carried out in hepatocyte endoplasmic reticulum and catalyzed by the system of oxidoreductases with the participation of cytochrome P_{450}. The reactions of the second group also proceed chiefly in liver with the participation of enzyme-transferases. Any of these reactions takes the steroid out of the sphere of biological action and they all pertain to the processes of steroid elimination. It can occur that in the process of AAS biotransformation, there appear metabolites whose activity can actually exceed the biological activity of the initial steroid. However, such a case is most likely an exception and applies to a limited number of AAS.

As stated above, the biological transformation of the AAS molecule leads to a rise in its hydrophilic properties which results in reducing the degree of its reabsorption by the epithelium of renal canals. In addition, glucuronides may be excreted from an organism along with bile and intestinal epithelium. Among the physical-chemical factors influencing AAS excretion, mainly with urine or bile, the molecular mass of steroids is of great importance. Steroid hormones having a molecular mass of less than 300 are eliminated from the organism chiefly with urine.

The velocities of excretion of various AAS from the human organism according to a steroid dose were studied in our laboratory. Initial experiments on volunteers investigated the time of 19-nortestosterone and norethandrolone excretion.[117] To identify AAS in urine the RID method was used. Figure 21 shows the results of determining norethandrolone in urine samples collected during different periods of time after oral ingestion of three steroids of different doses. As Figure 21 shows, 4 hours after norethandrolone ingestion the concentration of this steroid in urine reaches its maximum and its value is proportional to the dose used. Later, there occurs a reduction of hormone concentration which gradually approximates the urine samples of those who did not take the steroid. The character of the curves of steroid release after taking various doses is rather similar. The time of complete steroid excretion from the organism after a single ingestion takes from 48 to 72 hours. Analysis of the results of 19-nortestosterone

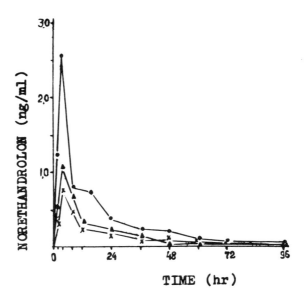

FIGURE 21.   Urinary excretion of norethandrolone after steroid ingestion in the following doses: 0.1 mg/kg wt (×—×), 0.2 mg/kg wt (Δ—Δ), 0.4 mg/kg wt (•—•).

elimination showed maximum concentration in urine to occur faster only 2 hours after ingestion. In other respects the character of the curves of AAS excretion was analogous to the results obtained in experiments with norethandrolone.

In subsequent experiments the concentration of 19-nortestosterone, methyl androstenediol, methandienone and norethandrolone in blood, saliva and urine of volunteers after a single steroid ingestion of 0.2 mg/kg was determined. Figure 22 gives the results of 19-nortestosterone and methandienone in human biological liquids.

These experiments demonstrate that the maximum concentration of AAS in blood and saliva occurs 2 hours after ingestion. Maximum concentration in urine for methandienone, 19-nortestosterone and norethandrolone occurred 2 to 4 hours postingestion, while it took 12 hours for methylandrostanediol. The maximum values of AAS concentration in blood are approximately 2 to 3 times higher than those in urine and 10 times higher than those in saliva. The differences in maximum values of various AAS in biological liquids within certain periods of time serve as evidence for the peculiarities of steroid metabolism. Therefore, the maximum concentrations of 19-nortestosterone and norethandrolone are about one order lower than the values for methandienone and methylandrostanediol and make up 0.3 to 0.5 ng/ml for saliva, 0.7 to 1.2 ng/ml for urine and 3.0 to 4.3 ng/ml for blood. These steroids with various intensities are involved in the processes of intracellular metabolism, which is reflected by the variation in concentrations in biological liquids.

Based on these preliminary experiments, more profound investigation on the time of elimination for 14 various AAS was carried out in our laboratory.[118] For this investigation we selected the most widespread of the AAS, the androstane, androstene and estrene series according to AAS classification given in Chapter 1. Table 21 gives the results of the concentration of these steroids in urine by means of the RIA method.

One can see that 11 of 14 steroids were excreted 2 hours after their introduction into the organism, with methandienone being excreted in the greatest concentration. Its concentration in urine considerably exceeds that of the other steroids. On the basis of the analysis of the curves of AAS elimination from an organism, one may come to a general conclusion that the concentrations of most of the investigated AAS in urine reach their maximum 2 to 8 hours after ingestion, with the exception of thiomesterone, stanozolol and methylandrostanediol whose maximum concentrations were observed 12 hours postingestion. The curve of stanozolol elimination showed a second maximum 44 to 60 hours postingestion, which is associated with a low velocity of release from the organism and is stipulated by the peculiarities of this steroid structure.[105] The time of complete elimination of all 14 investigated AAS from the organism after a single ingestion of 0.2 mg/kg does not exceed 72 hours.

By studying the time of elimination of AAS prolonged action (19-nortestosterone) it has been established that excretion of this steroid from the organism has

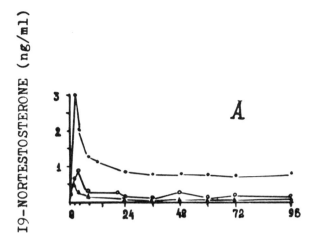

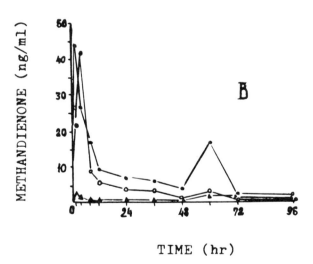

TIME (hr)

FIGURE 22. The concentration of 19-nortestosterone (A) and methandienone (B) in blood (•—•), saliva (Δ—Δ) and urine (○—○) after steroid ingestion at a dose of 0.2 mg/kg wt.

an undulating character and the high hormone concentrations can occur for a long period of time. To explain the reason for a prolonged delay of steroid action in an organism, the velocity of hormone transport from muscular depots to blood and the velocity of metabolism both in skeletal muscle and in blood and liver

TABLE 21
AAS Determination in Urine by RIA
2 Hours After Introduction into Organism

Steroid	Concentration in urine (ng/ml)
Androstane series	
Metenolone	16
Mesterolone	0
Oxandrolone	11
Oxymetholone	14
Stanozolol	18
Methylandrostanediol	0.4
Androstene series	
Methandienone	100
Methyltestosterone	8
Clostebol	0
Thiomesterone	5
Fluoxymesterone	0
Estrene series	
Norethandrolone	1.7
19-Nortestosterone	10

needs to be taken into consideration. The velocity of AAS metabolism is in many respects due to the spectrum and the capacity of the enzymic systems participating in steroid degradation as well as the transport systems involved (the principal factor regulating the time of the steroid staying in the organism). It should be noted that the time of AAS prolonged action and excretion from the human organism is strictly individual and may vary within large limits.

Besides the determination of the time of AAS release from the organism, it is also necessary to determine in what form they leave it — whether in a free form or in the form of conjugates with sulfuric or glucuronic acid. The determination of methandienone content in urine after a single ingestion showed that the ratio of free to conjugated fraction was 1:4. For 19-nortestosterone the ratio was 1:10; thus this steroid is excreted chiefly in a conjugated form.[119] The analysis of 10 various AAS showed that steroids of the estrene series were excreted mainly in the conjugated form. Steroids of the androstane series are, on the contrary, excreted in a free form. The steroids of androstene series take up an intermediate position; they may be removed both in a free or conjugated form.

Thus, the results given show the presence of enzymic systems in organisms which participate in AAS metabolism and their different distribution in tissues and liquids. Some pathways of metabolism and AAS elimination connected with the method of steroid introduction and the doses were revealed. All this makes it possible to determine the principal trends of AAS participation in the regulation of intracellular processes, which is discussed in the next chapter.

REFERENCES

1. *Nomenclature of Enzymes,* Academic Press, New York, 1979.
2. **Dorfman, R. L. and Ungar, F.,** *Metabolism of Steroid Hormones,* Academic Press, New York, 1965.
3. **Markin H. L. J., Ed.,** *Biochemistry of Steroid Hormones,* Blackwell Scientific Publications, Oxford, 1975.
4. **Mainwaring W. I. P.,** *The Mechanism of Action of Androgens,* Springer-Verlag, New York, 1977.
5. **Talalay, P. and Dobson, M. M.,** Purification and properties of a β-hydroxysteroid dehydrogenase, *J. Biol. Chem.,* 205, 823, 1953.
6. **Marcus, P. J. and Talalay, P.,** Induction and purification of α- and β-hydroxysteroid dehydrogenases, *J. Biol. Chem.,* 218, 661, 1956.
7. **Talalay, P. and Marcus, P. J.,** Specificity, kinetics and inhibition of α- and β-hydroxysteroid dehydrogenaes, *J. Biol. Chem.,* 218, 675, 1956.
8. **Roe, C. R. and Kaplan, N. O.,** Purification and substrate specificities of bacterial hydroxy-steroid dehydrogenases, *Biochemistry,* 8, 5093, 1969.
9. **MacDonald, J. A., Mahony, D. E., Meier, C. E., and Jellet, J. F.,** NAD-dependent 3α- and 12α-hydroxysteroid dehydrogenase activities from *Enbactorium lentum* ATCC N55559, *Biochim. Biophys. Acta,* 489, 466, 1977.
10. **Sih, C. J.,** Enzymatic mechanism of steroid hydroxylation, *Science,* 163, 1297, 1969.
11. **Gustafsson, J.-O. and Lisboa, B. P.,** Metabolism of C_{19} steroids in rat testis, *Eur. J. Biochem.,* 13, 554, 1970.
12. **Taurog, J. D., Moore, R. J., and Wilson, J. D.,** Partial characterization of the cytosol 3α-hydroxyl-steroid: NAD(P)⁺ oxidoreductase of rat ventral prostate, *Biochemistry,* 14, 810, 1975.
13. **Verhoeven, G., Heyns, W., and De Moor P.,** Interconversion between 17β-hydroxy-5α-androstan-3-one (5α-dihydrotestosterone) and 5α-androstane-3α,17β-diol in rat kidney: heterogeneity of 3α-hydroxysteroid oxidoreductases, *Eur. J. Biochem.,* 65, 565, 1976.
14. **Inano, H., Hayashi, S., and Tamaoki, S. I.,** Prostate 3α-hydroxysteroid dehydrogenase: its partial purification and properties, *J. Steroid Biochem.,* 8, 41, 1977.
15. **Peng, W. W., Wisner, J. R., and Warren, D. W.,** Testicular 3α-hydroxysteroid oxidoreduc-tase activity in the developing male rat, *Steroids,* 34, 101, 1979.
16. **Hastings, C. D., Brekke, J., Pruvis, K., Attramadal, A., and Hansson, V.,** Cofactor dependency of soluble 3α-hydroxysteroid oxidoreductases in rat testis, prostate and epididymis, *Endocrinology,* 107, 1762, 1980.
17. **Hastings, C. D., Brekke, J., Attramadal, A., and Hansson, V.,** Physicochemical characteri-zation of the soluble 3α-hydroxysteroid oxidoreductase in the rat testis and prostate, *Int. J. Androl.,* 3, 72, 1980.
18. **Baulieu, M. S.,** Androgen receptor in skeletal muscle, *J. Endocrinol.,* 65, 318, 1975.
19. **Lau, P., Layne, D. S., and Williamson, D. G.,** 3(17)α-Hydroxysteroid dehydrogenase of female rabbit kidney cytosol, *J. Biol. Chem.,* 257, 9444, 1982.
20. **Lau, P., Layne, D. S., and Williamson, D. G.,** Comparison of the multiple forms of the soluble 3(17)α-hydroxysteroid dehydrogenase of female rabbit kidney and liver, *J. Biol. Chem.,* 257, 9450, 1982.
21. **Maynard, P. V. and Cameron, E. H.,** Metabolism of androst-4-ene-3-17-dione by subcel-lular fractions of rat adrenal tissue with particular reference to microsomal C_{19} steroid 5α-reductase, *Biochem. J.,* 132, 183, 1973.
22. **Tamaoki, B. and Shikita, M.,** in *Steroid Dynamic,* Pincus, G. N. and Tait, J. F., Eds., Academic Press, New York, 1966, 393.
23. **Kruskemper, H.-L.,** *Anabolic Steroids,* Academic Press, New York, 1968.
24. **Hanquez-Laurent, Ch., De Lauzon, S., and Cittanova, N.,** Solubilization of 17α-hydroxy-steroid dehydrogenase from rat liver microsomes, *J. Steroid Biochem.,* 17, 647, 1982.

117

25. **Sweat, M. L., Samuels, L. T., and Lumry, R.,** Preparation and characterization of the enzyme which converts testosterone to androstendione, *J. Biol. Chem.,* 185, 75, 1950.
26. **Shefer, S., Hauser, S., and Mosbach, E. H.,** Studies on the biosynthesis of 5α-cholestan-3β-ol, *J. Biol. Chem.,* 341, 946, 1966.
27. **Davidson, S. J. and Talalay, P.,** Purification and mechanism of action of a steroid Δ^4-5β-dehydrogenase, *J. Biol. Chem.,* 241, 906, 1966.
28. **Collins, W. P., Konllapis, E. N., Bridges, C. E., and Sommervillo, I. F.,** Steroid metabolism in human prostatic tissue, *J. Steroid Biochem.,* 1, 195, 1970.
29. **Hudson, R. W., Moffitt, P. M., and Owens, W. A.,** Studies of the nuclear 5α-reductase of human prostatic tissue: comparison of enzyme activities in hyperplastic, malignant and normal tissues, *Can. J. Biochem. Cell. Biol.,* 61, 750, 1983.
30. **Habib, F. K., Tesdaje, A. L., Chishom, G. D., and Busuttil, A.,** Androgen metabolism in the epithelial and stromal components of the human hyperplastic prostate, *J. Endocrinol.,* 91, 23, 1981.
31. **Cowan, R. A., Cowan, S. A., Grant, J. K., and Elder, H. Y.,** Biochemical investigation of separated epithelium and stroma from benign hyperplastic tissue, *J. Endocrinol.,* 74, 111, 1977.
32. **Habib, F. K., Beynon, L., Chishoim, G. D., and Bustutil, A.,** The distribution of 5α-reductase and 3α(β)-hydroxysteroid dehydrogenase activity to the hyperplastic human prostate gland, *Steroids,* 41, 41, 1983.
33. **Orlowski, J., Bird, C. E., and Clark, A. F.,** Androgen 5α-reductase and 3α-hydroxysteroid dehydrogenase activities in ventral prostate epithelial and stromal cells from immature and mature rats, *J. Endocrinol.,* 99, 131, 1983.
34. **Clair, P., Patricot, M. C., Mothian, R., and Revol, R.,** Androgen metabolism in vitro by human leukocytes. Variations with sex and age, *J. Steroid Biochem.,* 20, 377, 1984.
35. **Grishanova, A. Yu., Mishin, V. W., and Lyakovich, V. V.,** Catalytic activity of cytochrome P-448 in native and reconstituted microsomal membranes, *Biochimiya (USSR),* 49, 1434, 1984.
36. **Capdevila, J., Saeki, Y., and Falck, J. R.,** The mechanistic plurality of cytochrome P_{450} and its biological ramification, *Xenobiotica,* 14, 186, 1984.
37. **Quengerich, F. P., Dannan, G. N., Wright, S. T., and Martin, M. V.,** Purification and characterization of liver microsomal cytochrome P-450, *Biochemistry,* 21, 6019, 1982.
38. **Sligar, S. G., Golb, M. H., and Heimbrock, D. C.,** Bio-organic chemistry and cytochrome P_{450} dependent catalysis, *Xenobiotica,* 14, 151, 1984.
39. **Boobis, A. R. and Davies, D. S.,** Human cytochromes P-450, *Xenobiotica,* 14, 151, 1984.
40. **Menard, R. M. and Purvis, J. L.,** Studies of cytochrome P-450 in testis microsomes, *Arch. Biochem. Biophy.,* 154, 8, 1973.
41. **Betz, G., Tsai, P., and Weakley, R.,** Heterogeneity of cytochrome P-450 in rat testis microsomes, *J. Biol. Chem.,* 251, 2839, 1976.
42. **Nakjin, S., Hall, P. F., and Onoda, M.,** Testicular microsomal cytochrome P-450 for C_{21} steroid side chain cleavage. Special and binding studies, *J. Biol. Chem.,* 256, 6134, 1981.
43. **Canick, J. A., Fox, C. D., and Callard, G. V.,** Studies on cytochrome P-450 dependent microsomal enzymes of testicular androgen and estrogen biosynthesis in a urodele amphibian Westurns, *J. Steroid Biochem.,* 21, 15, 1984.
44. **Ishii-Ohba, H., Matsumura, R., Inano, H., and Tamaoki, B.,** Contribution of cytochrome b_5 to androgen synthesis in rat testicular microsomes, *J. Biochem.,* 95, 335, 1984.
45. **Numazawa, M., Kimura, K., Nagaoka, M., and Ogata, M.,** Determination of aromatase activity involved in the formation of estriol with human placental microsomes and its kinetic properties, *J. Pharm.-Dyn.,* 7, 19, 1984.
46. **Akhar, M., Calder, M. D., Corina, D. L., and Wright, C. L.,** The status of oxygen atoms in removal of C_{19} in estrogen biosynthesis, *J. Chem. Soc. Chem. Commun.,* p. 129, 1981.
47. **Fishman, J. and Coto, J.,** Mechanism of estrogen biosynthesis: participation of multiple enzyme sites in placental aromatase hydroxylation, *J. Biol. Chem.,* 256, 4466, 1981.

48. **Thompson, J. E. and Sriteri, P. K.,** The involvement of human placental microsomal P_{450} in aromatization, *J. Biol. Chem.,* 249, 5373, 1979.

49. **Johnston, J. A., Wright, C. L., and Metcalf, B. W.,** Biochemical and endocrine properties of a mechanism-based inhibitor of aromatase, *Endocrinology,* 115, 776, 1984.

50. **Beusen, D. and Covey, D.,** Study of the role of Schiff base formation in the aromatization of 3-(^{18}O)-testosterone and 3,17-di-(^{18}O)-androstendione by human placental aromatase, *J. Steroid Biochem.,* 20, 931, 1984.

51. **Sheean L. and Meigs, R.,** The roles of NADH in the support of steroid aromatization by human placental microsomes, *Steroids,* 42, 77, 1983.

52. **Meigs, R. and Moorthy, K. B.,** The support of steroid aromatization by mitochondrial metabolic activities of the human placenta, *J. Steroid Biochem.,* 20, 11, 1984.

53. **Haaparanta, T., Glaumann, H., and Gustafsson, J.-Å.,** Characterization and endocrine regulation of the cytochrome P-450 dependent microsomal hydroxylation of 5-androstane-3,17-diol in the rat ventral prostate, *Endocrinology,* 114, 2293, 1984.

54. **Kühw-Velten, N., Bunse, T., Schüner, N., and Staib, W.,** Direct effect of androgens on progesterone binding and metabolism in rat testis microsomes, *Hoppe-Seyler's Z. Physiol. Chem.,* 365, 773, 1984.

55. **Gower, D. B.,** Properties and subcellular location of enzymes involved in steroidogenesis (and the role of cytochrome P-450), in *Biochemistry of Steroid Hormones,* Makin, H. L., Ed., Blackwell Scientific Publications, Oxford, 1975, 105.

56. **Payne, A. H. and Singer, S. S.,** The role of steroid sulfatase and sulphotransferase enzymes in metabolism of C_{21} and C_{19} steroids, in *Steroid Biochemistry,* Hobkirk, R., Ed., CRC Press, Boca Raton, FL, 1979, 1.

57. **Prescott, L. F.,** Drug conjugation in clinical toxicology, *Biochem. Soc. Trans.,* 12, 96, 1984.

58. **Bailey-Wood, R., Dodgson, K., and Rose, F. A.,** Purification and properties of two adenosine-5'-phosphosulphate sulphohydrolases from rat liver and their possible role in the degradation of 3'-phosphoadenosine-5'-phosphosulphate, *Biochim. Biophys. Acta,* 220, 284, 1970.

59. **Gower, D. B.,** Unsaturated C_{19} steroids. A review of their chemistry, biochemistry and possible physiological role, *J. Steroid Biochem.,* 3, 45, 1972.

60. **Cooke, G. M., Ferguson, S. E., Rytina, E., and Gower, D. B.,** Properties of porcine liver and testicular steroid sulphotransferases: reaction conditions and influence of naturally occurring steroid and steroid sulphates, *J. Steroid Biochem.,* 19, 1103, 1983.

61. **Ryan, R. A. and Carrol, J.,** Studies in a 3β-hydroxysteroid sulphotransferase from rat liver, *Biochim. Biophys. Acta,* 429, 392, 1979.

62. **Nose, Y. and Lipmann, F.,** Separation of steroid sulphokinase, *J. Biol. Chem.,* 233, 1348, 1958.

63. **Fish, D. E., Cooke, G. M., and Grower, D. B.,** Investigation into the sulpho conjugation of 5α-androst-16-en-3β-ol by porcine liver, *FEBS Lett.,* 117, 2832, 1980.

64. **Cooke, G. M., Ferguson, S. E., Rytina, F., and Gower, D. B.,** Properties of porcine liver and testicular steroid sulphotransferases: reaction conditions and influence of naturally occurring steroids and steroid sulphates, *J. Steroid Biochem.,* 19, 403, 1983.

65. **Cooke, G. M. and Gower, D. B.,** The submicrosomal distribution in rat and boar testis of some enzymes involved in androgen and 16-androstene biosynthesis, *Biochim. Biophys. Acta,* 498, 265, 1977.

66. **Cooke, G. M. and Gower, D. B.,** Investigation into the possible effects of naturally occurring steroids on biosynthesis of 16-androstanes and androgens in microsomes of boar testis, *J. Endocrinol.,* 88, 409, 1981.

67. **Nishikawa, T. and Strott, O.,** Unconjugated and sulphoconjugated steroids in plasma and zones of the adrenal cortex of the guinea pig, *Steroids,* 41, 105, 1983.

68. **Dutton, G. J.,** Introduction to biological functions of glucuronidation, in *Glucuronidation of Drugs and Other Compounds,* Dutton, G. J., Ed., CRC Press, Boca Raton, FL, 1980, 3.

69. **Keppen, B. and Dalgaard L.,** Assay for β-glucuronidase utilizing headspace gas chromatography, *Anal. Biochem.,* 136, 272, 1984.
70. **Burchell, B.,** Substrate specificity and properties of urine diphosphate glucuronyl transferase purified to apparent homogeneity from phenobarbital-treated rat liver, *Biochem J.,* 173, 749, 1978.
71. **Rao, G. S., Haueter, G., Rao, M. L., and Breuer, H.,** Steroid glucuronosyl transferase of rat liver, *Biochem. J.,* 162, 5454, 1977.
72. **Matsui, M., Nagao, F., and Aoyagi, S.,** Strain differences in rat liver UDP glucuronosyl transferase activity towards androsterone, *Biochem. J.,* 179, 483, 1979.
73. **Matsui, M. and Watanade, H. K.,** Classification and genetic expression of Wistar rats with high and low hepatic microsomal UDP glucuronosyl transferase activity towards androsterone, *Biochem. J.,* 202, 171, 1982.
74. **Weatherill, P. J. and Burchell, B.,** The separation and purification of rat liver UDP-glucuronyl transferase activities towards testosterone and oestrone, *Biochem. J.,* 189, 377, 1980.
75. **Mackenzie, P. J. and Owens, J. S.,** Purification of a form of mouse liver UDP glucuronosyl transferase which glucuronidate androgens, *J. Steroid Biochem.,* 19, 1097, 1983.
76. **Schweider, G., French, A., Bullack, L., and Bardin, C. W.,** Absence of androgen stimulation of hepatic steroid sulfatase in the female rat, *Endocrinology,* 89, 308, 1971.
77. **Fishman, J., Bradlow, H. L., Zumoff, B., Hellman, L., and Gallagher, T. F.,** Further studies of the metabolism of oestradiol in man, *Acta Endocrinol.,* 37, 57, 1961.
78. **Kellie, A. E.,** The extraction and hydrolysis of steroid monoglucuronides, *Biochem. J.,* 100, 631, 1966.
79. **Krebs, E. G. and Beavo, T. A.,** Phosphorylation-dephosphorylation of enzymes, *Annu. Rev. Biochem.,* 48, 923, 1979.
80. **Von Will, H.,** Zur Rolle von Proteinphosphorylierungen in der Zellregulation, *Dt. Gesundh. Wesen.,* 37, 201, 1983.
81. **Kuo, J. F., Andersson, R. G., Weise, B. C., Mackerleva, L., Solomonsson, J., and Brackett, N. L.,** Calcium-dependent protein kinase: widespread occurrence in various tissues and phyla of the animal kingdom and comparison of effects of phospholipid, calmodulin and trifluoperazine, *Proc. Natl. Acad. Sci. USA,* 77, 7039, 1980.
82. **Kennedy, M. B. and Greengard, P.,** Two calcium/calmodulin-dependent protein kinases which are highly concentrated in brain, phosphorylate protein 1 at distinct sites, *Proc. Natl. Acad. Sci. USA,* 78, 1293, 1981.
83. **Glebov, R. N.,** AMP and Ca-dependent phosphorylation of functional-significant proteins in presynoptical structures, *Uspechi Sov. Biol. (USSR),* 91, 433, 1981.
84. **Brostrom, C. O. and Wolf, D. J.,** Properties and function of calmodulin, *Biochem. Pharmacol.,* 30, 1395, 1981.
85. **Antoniw, J. F. and Cohen, R.,** Separation of phosphorylase kinase phosphatase from rabbit skeletal muscle, *Eur. J. Biochem.,* 68, 45, 1976.
86. **Khandelwal, R. L. and Zinman, S. M.,** The presence of heat-stable activator of phosphoprotein phosphatase for the dephosphorylation of phosphorylated histone in rabbit liver, *Biochem. Biophys. Res. Commun.,* 82, 1340, 1978.
87. **Kinohara, N., Usui, H., Imaru, M., Imaoka, T., and Takeda, M.,** A survey of multiple phosphoprotein phosphatase in cytosol from rat tissues and erythrocytes, *J. Biochem.,* 91, 177, 1982.
88. **Clari, G., Donella, A., Pinna, B. A., and Maret, V.,** Further characterization of mitochondrial protein phosphatase, *Arch. Biochem. Biophys.,* 166, 318, 1975.
89. **Olson, M. O. J. and Guetzow, K. A.,** Nuclear phosphoprotein phosphatase from Novikoff hepatoma and rat liver: characterization and partial purification, *Biochim. Biophys. Acta,* 526, 174, 1978.
90. **Dziembor-Guszkiewsz, E., Kis, S., Kuciel, R., Pilch, P., Sashenko, L. P., Wasylewska, E.,**

and Ostrowski, W., Distribution and some properties of phosphoprotein phosphatase activity in rat liver chromatin, *Biologia,* 38, 305, 1978.

91. **Ingebritsen, T. S. and Cohen, P.,** The protein phosphatases involved in cellular regulation. I. Classification and substrate specificities, *Eur. J. Biochem.,* 132, 255, 1983.

92. **Foulkes, J. G., Strada, S. J., Henderson, R. J., and Cohen, P.,** A kinetic analysis of the effects of inhibitor-1 and inhibitor-2 in activity of protein phosphatase-1, *Eur. J. Biochem.,* 132, 309, 1983.

93. **Chon, M. W., Tan, E. L., and Yang, C. S.,** Nuclear phosphoprotein phosphatase from calf liver, *Biochim. Biophys. Acta,* 56, 49, 1979.

94. **Shimazu, T.,** Liver phosphorylase phosphatase, *Mol. Cell Biochem.,* 49, 3, 1982.

95. **Imooka, T., Imazu, M., Usui, H., Kinohara, N., and Takeda, M.,** Isolation of an inactive component from pig heart phosphoprotein phosphatase and reassociation with an active component, *J. Biol. Chem.,* 258, 1526, 1983.

96. **Szeszak, F. and Pinna, L. A.,** Protein phosphatase from liver nuclei, *Biol. Cell Biochem.,* 32, 13, 1980.

97. **Auricchio, F., Migliaccio, A., and Rotondi, A.,** Inactivation of oestrogen receptor in vitro by nuclear dephosphorylation, *Biochem. J.,* 194, 569, 1981.

98. **Auricchio, F., Migliaccio, A., Castoria, S., Lastoria, S., and Rotondi, A.,** Evidence that in vivo estradiol receptor translocated into nuclei is dephosphorylated and released into cytoplasm, *Biochem. Biophys. Res. Commun.,* 106, 149, 1982.

99. **Auricchio, F., Migliaccio, A., Castoria, G., Rotondi, A., and Lastoria, S.,** Direct evidence of in vitro phosphorylation-dephosphorylation of the estradiol-17β, *J. Steroid Biochem.,* 20, 31, 1984.

100. **Templeton, J. F. and Kim, R.,** Metabolism of 17β-hydroxy-2α-methyl-5α-androstan-3-one in the rabbit, *Steroids,* 19, 371, 1977.

101. **Gerhards, E., Kolb, K. H., and Schulze, P. E.,** Zum Stoffwechsel von 17β-Acetoxy-1-methyl-Δ¹-5α-androsteron-3 (Methenolon-acetat) beim Menschen, *Hoppe-Seyler Z. Physiol. Chem.,* 342, 40, 1965.

102. **Adkihary, P. M. and Harkness, R. A.,** Use of carbon skeleton chromatography for the detection of steroid drug metabolisms, *Acta Endocrinol.,* 67, 721, 1971.

103. **Pokrovsky, B. V.,** Metabolism in vivo of dehydromethyltestosterone (methanandrostenolone) and methyltestosterone in rats tissues, *Probl. Endocrinol.,* 14, 369, 1968.

104. **Mac Donald, B. S., Sykes, P. J., Adhikary, P. M., and Harkness, R. A.,** The identification of 17α-hydroxy-17β-methylandrosta-1,4-dien-3-one as a metabolite of 17β-hydroxy-17α-methylandrosta-1,4-dien-3-one in man, *Biochem. J.,* 122, 26 P, 1971.

105. **Ward, R. J., Lawson, A. M., and Shackleton, C. H. L.,** Screening by gas chromatography-mass-spectrometry for metabolites of five commonly used steroid drugs, in *Mass Spectrometry in Drug Metabolism,* Frigerio, A. and Chisalbert, E. L., Eds., Plenum Press, New York, 1977, 465.

106. **Duerbeck, J., Scheulen, B., and Telin, B.,** Gas chromatography and capillary column gas chromatography-mass spectrometry determination of synthetic anabolic steroid, *J. Chromatogr. Sci.,* 21, 405, 1983.

107. **Ward, R. J., Lawson, A. M., and Schakleton, C. H. L.,** Metabolism of anabolic steroid drugs in man and the marmoset monkey *(Callithrix jacchus),* nilevar and orabolin, *J. Steroid Biochem.,* 8, 1057, 1977.

108. **Stelle, J. W., Boux, L. J., and Audette, R. C.,** Anabolic steroids, *Xenobiotica,* 11, 103, 1981.

109. **Kupfer, D. and Peets, L. M.,** Characteristics of estrogen-mediated inhibition of cortisol ring A reduction by liver microsomes, *Arch. Biochem. Biophys.,* 121, 392, 1967.

110. **Weintraub, H., Vincent, F., Baulieu, E. E., and Alfsen, A.,** Interaction of steroids with *Pseudomonas testosteroni* 3-oxo-steroid Δ⁴-Δ⁵-isomerase, *Biochemistry,* 16, 5045, 1977.

111. **Templeton, J. F. and Jackson, Ch. C.,** Metabolism of 17α-methyl-testosterone in the rabbit: C-6 and C-16 hydroxylated metabolites, *Steroids,* 42, 115, 1983.

112. **Härkonen, P.,** Androgenic control of glycolysis, the pentose cycle and pyruvate dehydrogenase in the rat ventral prostate, *J. Steroid Biochem.,* 14, 1075, 1981.
113. **Gribbin, H. R. and Flavell Matts, S. G.,** Mode of action and use of anabolic steroids, *Bioph. J. Clin. Pract.,* 30, 3, 1976.
114. **James, K. C., Nicholls, P. J., and Roberts, M.,** Biological half-lives of 4-^{14}C-testosterone and some of its esters after injection into the rat, *J. Pharm. Pharmacol.,* 21, 24, 1969.
115. **Soloviev, V. N., Firsov, A. A., and Filov, V. A.,** *Pharmacokinetics,* Medicine, Moscow, 1980.
116. **Williams, R. T.,** *Detoxication Mechanisms. The Metabolism and Detoxication of Drugs, Toxic Substances and Other Organic Compounds,* John Wiley & Sons, New York, 1960.
117. **Prijatkin, S. A., Morosov, V. I., and Garnovsky, A. V.,** Investigation on various anabolic steroids excreting from organism, in *Medical and Doping Control of Athletes,* Research Institute of Physical Culture, Leningrad, 1981, 64.
118. **Prijatkin, S. A. and Garnovsky, A. V.,** Investigation on anabolic steroids excretion from organism, *Sci. Rev. Tartu Univ.,* 619, 101, 1983.
119. **Litvinova, V. N.,** Chemical structures of anabolic steroids on gas chromatograph-mass-spectrometer and some ways of biosamples preparation for the analysis, in *Medical and Doping Control of Athletes,* Research Institute of Physical Culture, Leningrad, 1981, 103.

Chapter 7

THE ROLE OF AAS IN REGULATION OF METABOLISM IN NORM AND PATHOLOGY AND THEIR USE IN MEDICINE AND CATTLE BREEDING

The problems associated with the use of AAS in the regulation of intracellular metabolism in various tissues and by different states of an organism occupy one of the central places in the problem of studying the mechanisms of steroid hormone action. This occurs for the simple reason that, on the one hand, the basic effect of AAS on an organism is associated with anabolic processes in the cell, while on the other hand and in many cases AAS also retain an androgenic action and participate in metabolic reactions together or in place of endogenous androgens. These data, as well as some others, give every reason to suppose that AAS can take an active part in the regulation of many reactions of intracellular metabolism and exert a versatile influence on the content of various endogenous hormones and in this way specifically regulate metabolic processes in the cell. The versatility of the action of AAS in an organism is confirmed by a large number of effects which are demonstrated by a systematic use of such hormones. Among them one can mention the growth of the body and individual organ weight, the rise in concentration of separate substances, and the increase in the activity of a series of enzymes.

Additionally, changes in human behavior were demonstrated after a prolonged intake of AAS. A number of effects of AAS are associated with the activities of the sex glands and their involvement with sexual behavior. Some other effects of these hormones may be attributed, to a greater degree, to social behavior where they are manifested in a display of aggressive behavior. Often they are used within the context of sports competition. In a number of cases the effects of AAS on an organism prove to be exaggerated and are not adequate to their real possibilities. One should carefully regard all the investigations where AAS are used so as to be able to ascertain how these hormones are involved in the mechanisms of intracellular regulation of metabolic processes in an organism.

The study of the effect of various AAS on nitrogen delay in organisms and possible changes in nitrogen balance showed that this process was strictly determined and it could not exceed a certain value. The delay of nitrogen in a human organism did not exceed 23% and is independent of sex, age, nutrition, and physical exercise. A wide range of AAS doses used (2.5 to 150 mg/ day) had no effect on the change of the values of nitrogen delay in the organism either. It turned out that human anabolic potential could not exceed the value by more than 23% and the use of AAS with various chemical structures did not cause its subsequent rise. It is rather characteristic that to obtain the highest possible response, that is the value of nitrogen delay by 23%, it is not obligatory to use high doses of steroids. Such an effect is achieved with doses of 2.5 mg/day and higher doses do not promote the development of anabolic effects.

The possibility of an increase in human body weight under the influence of AAS use is shown in a series of investigations. It is associated with the delay of both nitrogen and water.[1-7] On the other hand, it has been established that body weight growth by AAS application may be achieved only on the basis of sufficiently providing the organism with an indispensable quantity of valuable protein.[8] Active AAS participation in the regulation of intracellular metabolism causes considerable changes in the utilization of food substances in an organism and it may favor a more perfect assimilation of various vegetable proteins as well.[9] It should be noted that there are some observations in which no change in body weight, after prolonged AAS ingestion (for 8 to 16 weeks), was seen.[10-12]

When examining the principal effects of AAS on intracellular metabolism it is necessary to distinguish those that include the widest range of both separate biochemical reactions and entire metabolic cycles. Except for an active part in the regulation of protein synthesis, which is discussed in Chapter 5, the action of AAS is associated with the regulation of carbohydrate, lipid, and mineral metabolism, as well as with the regulation of the activity of a number of endogenic glands. Thus, the presence of two mechanisms of AAS action in an organism both directly and by means of the endocrine system considerably enlarges the list of metabolic processes which make up a regulated function of this group of steroid hormones.

The changes observed in metabolism under the influence of AAS mainly occur in liver, skeletal muscles, heart and sex organs.

AAS participation in the regulation of carbohydrate metabolism in an organism was seen in the same biochemical reactions which were controlled by endogenic androgens. The influence of testosterone on the delay of glucose in skeletal muscle may be considered to be an example.[13] It has been established that 3.5 hours after testosterone-propionate injection, the content of glucose in skeletal muscles is considerably increased and it remains at a high level during the subsequent 72 hours. 5-Dihydrotestosterone and AAS-fluoroxymesterone also possess analogous action. The level of the increase of glucose content under the influence of AAS is different in various skeletal muscles according to their morphological characteristics and functional profile. The molecular mechanism of the action of AAS concerning the exchange of glucose is still vague; however it is associated with the formation of the hormone-receptor complex and is carried out with the participation of androgen receptors. Other steroid hormones, such as 17β-estradiol and corticosterone, do not exert an appreciable influence on the delay of glucose in skeletal muscles. While examining the effect of AAS on the content of glucose in blood, it is necessary to note that 17-alkylated AAS allow the reduction of a normal level of glucose to low values. The other AAS manifest such an action only through the presence of a high content of glucose in blood, which is observed in persons having diabetes or having a predisposition to it.[14,15] In these cases the sensitivity of tissues to insulin, specifically liver, is increased under the influence of AAS. After ingestion of 17-alkylated AAS the degree of insulin inactivation in liver changes, the level of glucose in blood is reduced, and a state of hypoglycemia gradually develops. This can be seen in outward symptoms of human behavior. There appear such symptoms as perspiration, shivering, headache, and giddiness, which cease after eating. Under these conditions, when the level of glucose in blood is low, the organism may use its reserve fat as a source of energy. In the blood of humans who take AAS, parallel with the decrease in the level of blood glucose, an increase in free fatty acid concentration is observed and is associated with a metabolic alteration in the liver.[16] The development of a hypoglycemic state in humans who take AAS is evident from the high content of fatty acids in blood.

At present there is much data concerning the possible action of AAS on lipid metabolism.[17,18] AAS increase the concentration of cholesterol and triglycerides in blood. Although many processes in the development of arteriosclerosis are still unknown, a high level of cholesterol in blood may be considered as an important factor in the process of forming arteriosclerosed yellow plaque on the inner layers of the arterial wall. Cholesterol and other lipids are transported in human and animal organisms by special carriers called plasma lipoproteins. It has been established that lipoproteins are divided into three classes: chylomicrons, lipoproteins of a very low density (LPLD) and lipoproteins of a high density (LPHD). Chylomicrons are formed in epithelial cells of the small intestine in the process of fat adsorption. They serve as a triglyceride transport form of food origin and other tissues. LPLD are formed in the liver and their function is associated with the transport of endogenic (synthesized in liver) triglycerides. LPLD are synthesized in blood and are considered to be a principal form of cholesterol transport which is carried with food or synthesized in the organism. The function of LPHD is associated with a return transport of cholesterol from peripheral tissues to the liver for a subsequent repeated involvement into the complex with LPLD or oxidation into gallic acids and excretion from the organism with bile. By studying the transport of lipids to the cell, a direct interaction of chylomicrons and LPLD with the enzyme lipoprotein lipase, which was localized in the wall of the capillaries of fatty tissue, heart muscle, spleen, kidneys, diaphragm and other tissues, has been established. As a result of lipoprotein lipase action on triglycerides of chylomicrons and LPLD, monoglycerides and fatty acids are formed. They penetrate tissues and cells and in the process of diffusion become involved in intracellular metabolism. Study of the mechanism of LPLD cholesterin transport to peripheral tissues allowed Goldstein and Brown to formulate a hypothesis of LPLD receptor interaction with the cell.[19] According to this hypothesis LPLD possess a high content of apoprotein B which may be bound by specific receptors of protein and which are placed on the surface of cells of parenchymous and connective tissues. After the formation of such a complex (LPSD-cell) there occurs a gradual pinocytosis of the complex inside the cell where successive metabolic transformations of lipoprotein particles under the action of lysosomal enzymes are accomplished.[20]

Cholesterol remains in the cell and participates in various reactions of intracellular metabolism. A receptor placed on the surface of the cell may bind one LPLD. The total number of receptors that interact with LPLD in various tissues ranges from 15,000 to 60,000. The whole process of LPLD interaction with the cell and subsequent splitting of the lipoprotein complex occurs within 3 min, which allows estimation of the transport of cholesterol by blood.

According to Goldstein and Brown's hypothesis, a specific receptor interaction of LPLD with a cell with a subsequent hydrolysis of the lipoprotein complex inside the cell may be the main factor regulating a normal level of cholesterol in the blood.[21] Another factor involved in the regulation of the level of cholesterol in an organism is associated with the unique ability of LPLD to accept cholesterol from the membrane of parenchymous and connective tissue of cells and transport it to the liver for subsequent excretion from the organism.

The content of cholesterol in an organism depends not only on a considerable amount of LPLD delivered to peripheral tissues, but also on the quantity of LPLD which is taken away from these tissues. In the presence of balance in these processes, the level of cholesterol in an organism remains constant. An increase in the amount of LPLD leads to the intensification of cholesterol transport to the cells of peripheral tissues, which creates the risk of developing cholesterol deposits. A number of subsequent investigations have established that a high LPLD concentration increases the possibility of the appearance of arteriosclerosis, while a high LPHD concentration decreases the possibility of developing this disease.

Thus, according to the profile of lipoprotein complexes one may evaluate to some extent the process of developing arteriosclerosis in an organism. The application of AAS rapidly and considerably reduces the concentration of LPHD in the blood. If the content of LPHD in the blood of a healthy human being makes up 40 to 60 mg/dl, then after AAS intake these values make up only 5 to 10 mg/dl,[17,22,23] which considerably increases the possibility of formation of cholesterol deposits. It may create a predisposition for the development of arteriosclerosis.

The influence of AAS on the nervous and endocrine systems was investigated. It was manifested in an increase in the production of a number of hypothalamic and hypophyseal hormones which led to a rise in the concentration of hormones in the blood and tissues. The effect of AAS on metabolism in some organs and tissues may be manifested under the action of other hormones. Under the influence of hormones from the adrenal cortex, some alterations in the regulation of electrolyte exchange occur. It may be reflected by the activity of the cardiovascular system and lead to a rise in blood pressure. Aldosterone, cortisol, and corticosterone participate in the regulation of water electrolyte exchange. The action of aldosterone is carried out mainly at the level of renal epithelium. As for cortisol and corticosterone, they regulate the transport of ions through the cellular membrane. The participation of the Na-K pump in an active Na excretion from the cell and K transport to the cell is closely associated energy metabolism and regulated by Na-K-ATP-ase. The dependence of this enzyme activity on the presence of adrenocortical hormones has been shown in a number of works.[24,25]

The occurrence of hypercortisolemia, associated with an increase in the cortisol level in blood, is widespread after AAS ingestion.[26] It has been observed that under the influence of some AAS, the velocity of 17-oxosteroid excretion from an organism is considerably reduced. 17α-Methyl-19-nortestosterone, 17α-ethyl-19-nortestosterone, and methandienone also possess such a pronounced effect. The other AAS, 19-nortestosterone-phenylpropionate and methenolone, had virtually no influence on the velocity of 17-oxosteroid excretion.[27]

By studying the half-life of cortisol it has been established that in the presence of AAS, this hormone is excreted from an organism considerably slower. It is connected with a reduction in the velocity of cortisol inactivation in the liver. It has also been established that AAS are able to increase the level of transcortin in blood and increase the amount of bound cortisol. The reason for cortisol delay is probably due to the change in velocity of a number of enzyme reactions occurring in the liver. One is an AAS competitor with cortisol for the enzyme 3β-hydroxysteroid dehydrogenase, while another is also linked with competition for glucuronic acid during the formation of conjugates.[28] When discussing a possible effect of AAS on the enzyme 3β-hydroxysteroid dehydrogenase, it should be taken into consideration that the group of oral AAS-17α-alkylated steroids strongly inhibits the activity of this enzyme. This is reflected by the velocity of cortisol catabolism and prolongs the time of its presence in an organism. The high concentration of cortisol influences different parts of intracellular metabolism and leads to alterations in carbohydrate turnover in the liver. Under the action of cortisol, release of glucose from liver increases and glycogenesis and glyconeogenesis from amino acids increase. In the process of glyconeogenesis there occurs a rise in the activity of several enzymes localized in the liver: glucoso-6-phosphatases, aminotransferases, pyruvate carboxylase and glycogen synthase. The action of cortisol in peripheral tissues leads to a reduction in the velocity of amino acid involvement in protein synthesis and moreover intensifies its use as a substrate of glyconeogenesis. The intensification of the metabolism of nucleic acids and proteins in the liver in the presence of a high cortisol concentration may also be noted. A mobilizing effect of hormones on lipid metabolism, which is accompanied by the release of free fatty acids, is also seen. The diversity of the effect of cortisol on metabolism in the liver and peripheral organs should be taken into account. Among other effects of cortisol, one may also distinguish a delay of water and electrolytes. In certain cases it may cause some alterations in the cardiovascular system and be the reason for the observed rise in blood pressure. Thus, the list of possible effects of AAS on metabolism by a change in the cortisol degradation velocity in the liver is rather extensive, and according to these consequences and changes in metabolism, these collateral effects may considerably influence the functional state of separate organism systems. They concern hypercalcemia which can lead to a delay in calcium excretion from the organism, which is accompanied by calcium deposits forming in the joints as well as the formation of stones in the kidney and the disturbance of many other processes in various tissues.

In recent years AAS have been used on a large scale in clinical medicine, although in many cases their specific mechanism of action and possible collateral effects are out of sight of the investigators. It has been shown that the action of AAS on the cardiovascular system may be manifested in several directions. The total increase in arterial blood circulation, especially in the region of the coronary arteries and the vessels of the central nervous system, has been shown.[18] An increase in the contractile proteins of heart muscle and an increase in general tone of the heart and vessels were noted. A decrease in the level of cholesterol and phospholipids in blood was also observed. As a result of nandrolone-phenylpropionate (15 to 30 mg/day for 3 weeks) use, a positive effect was observed in patients with chronic coronary heart disease.[29,30] Out of 159 patients a painful syndrome disappeared in 101, was reduced in 32, and did not change in 25. Symptoms of myocardial ischemia displayed by electrocardiograph disappeared in 18 patients; 124 patients with rheumatic heart disease and arteriosclerosis cardiosclerosis with blood circulation insufficiency were observed. Methandrostenolone application led to a reduction in the syndrome of hypodynamia.[31] It was shown that 10 mg/day of ethylestrenol or stanozolol promotes the intensification of lipid metabolism and leads to fat mobilization and an increase in fibrinolytic activity in human blood. After taking therapeutic doses of AAS, an increase in fibrinolytic activity led to widespread use of these hormones for the purpose of treating heart ischemia.[16,18,32] After myocardial infarction, a reduction of fibrinolysis was seen and application of this group of steroids for increasing the activity of this system is possible.

AAS are widely used for the purpose of treating ulcerous diseases of the stomach and duodenum.[33,34] The therapeutic action of these hormones is distinctly manifested in ulcer cicatrication and the reduction of disturbed protein metabolism. As for chronic gastritis and enterocolitis, AAS improves the metabolism of ventricle epithelium and exerts a favorable influence on the regulation of gastric juice acidity.[35] In nephrology, AAS are used for an increase of nitrogenous substances caused by acute renal insufficiency. These hormones exert a favorable influence on kidney diseases proceeding with hypoproteinemia phenomena. According to the observations of some physiologists, AAS (in combination with special tuberculostatical preparations) exert a therapeutic effect for the treatment of initial and chronic forms of pulmonary tuberculosis.[36,37] An improvement in general state, appetite, reduction of asthenia symptoms, and body mass growth in patients was observed during AAS therapeutics. AAS have also found applications in hematology for treating various forms of anemia (hypo- and aplastic forms) especially in women. The differences in androgenic status of males and females have been seen by the content of fat which closely correlates with the level of androgens in the organism. The lower the concentration of androgens, the larger the mass of reserve fat and the less intensive is its expenditure. A low level of androgens also leads to the deceleration of erythropoiesis, which is reflected by the amount of erythrocytes and in their basic physical-chemical properties.[38] The application of therapeutic doses of androgens and AAS for treatment of various forms of anemias, especially in women, leads to an increase in the velocity of erythropoiesis, an increase in the amount of erythrocytes, and an increase in the content of hemoglobin.[39] Intensification of the synthesis of erythropoiesis in the kidneys is the basis for the metabolic effects of steroids. The mechanism of hormonal action is due to a receptor apparatus and is associated with the intensification of the synthesis of erythropoiesis and β-glucuronidase enzyme. Some attempts have been made to use AAS for treating the insufficiency of marrow function linked with aplastic anemia as well as for anemia by renal insufficiency. In a number of cases, during prolonged application of therapeutic doses of oxymetholone, some positive results for hematocrit and the content of hemoglobin were obtained.[40] It turned out that the most essential medical effect was obtained in patients suffering from marrow hypoplasia[41] and microfibrolysis.[42] However it should be noted that in the use of AAS in treating various forms of anemias, there remain many problems concerning hormone dosage, therapeutic periods, and, of course, the mechanism of their action. It can occur that therapeutic doses of AAS do not give a favorable effect for some forms of anemia.[43]

The use of 17α-alkylated AAS for treating hereditary dropsy led, in most cases, to positive results, and it had rather wide confirmation.[44,45] It was shown that this group of steroids caused an increase in the content of some glycoproteins such as haptoglobin, plasminogen, fibrinogen and ceruloplasmin in blood.[46,47] In AAS traumatology, the accumulation of calcium, phosphorus and sulfur is widely used for the intensification of protein synthesis in the basic substance of bone for treating fractures which dot not knit for a long time and after a number of osseous-plastic operations.[48,49] The use of AAS for treating various endocrine diseases has shown that the therapeutic effects of these steroids are specific for the treatment of diabetes, toxic goiter, hormonal spondylopathies, and hypothyrosis.[16] It should be noted that the use of AAS for treating various diseases did not always lead to positive results. Some data show that in some cases, these steroid hormones do not exert any favorable action, or sometimes it is of short duration.[50—53]

The experience of using AAS in clinical medicine shows that parallel to certain medicinal effects AAS, primarily 17α-alkylated AAS, cause a number of side effects which in some cases are undesirable and threatening to human health. There also exist some side effects of AAS caused by their physiological action. They occur in the localities which are undesirable for a healthy organism. One may note a virilization which is possible and necessary for men and which is extremely undesirable for women and children.

Among other diseases which are revealed by systematic AAS use, it is necessary to point out the possibility of the development of testicular tumors in male sex organs. An inhibiting effect of these steroids on the secretion of gonadotropin, as well as the size of testicles and spermatogenesis, is convincingly shown in experiments on both humans and animals.

Another factor which indicates a possible participation of AAS in the development of oncologic diseases in humans is due to the disturbance of the hormonal status in the organism. After AAS use, the production of many endogenic hormones, such as testosterone, gonadotropins, growth hormone, adrenocorticotropin and some others, is sharply reduced.[54]

The disturbance of hormonal regulation is considerably reflected by intracellular metabolism and leads to the following phenomenon: in a number of organs some cells become out of control and then become a potential area for the development of a series of oncologic diseases.[55]

The effect of AAS on liver metabolism is associated primarily with steroid biotransformations and their conversion into substances which are extracted from the organism. In the process of steroid biotransformation, some alterations of the substances containing nitrogen in liver occur. This may be seen through the accumulation of bilirubin and a change in aminotransferase activity. The increase in aminotransferase activity in blood may only be seen by the most sensitive tests which testify to some disturbance in the metabolism of substances containing nitrogen in the liver. By using 17α-alkylated and other oral AAS, an increase in the level of bilirubin and aminotransferase activity is seen and is dependent on the steroid dosage.

Prolonged application of AAS causes metabolic disturbances in the liver and leads to the appearance of grave pathological alterations which may be revealed in the form of progressive cholecystitis and jaundice.[56] We have information that shows that prolonged use of 17α-alkylated AAS may cause the development of tumors in the liver, and in some cases hepatomas and other forms of malignant neoplasms have been observed.[57] Although in the case of AAS application the pathogenesis of these diseases remains vague, there exist some suppositions about a possible accumulation of hepatocytes in the liver vein spaces which impedes blood circulation and leads to the accumulation of carcinogenic metabolites.[58—60]

The information on the development of hepatitis and hepatomas in the liver in those who took AAS appears to be rather threatening. Originally, such facts were established in patients who had various forms of anemias and went through a course of medical treatment using AAS. Then there appeared some reports on the possibility of developing oncologic diseases in the course of AAS use.[61] AAS may also exert considerable influence on the development of heart and blood vessel diseases. The application of this group of steroids may lead to the appearance of arteriosclerotic symptoms, increased blood pressure, alterations in the process of coagulation, and an increase in blood clot formation. In the end it raises the risk of a grave disturbance in cardiovascular system activity.[17,62]

In recent years a new trend in endocrinology has begun to develop in clinical medicine. It is concerned with the development of a number of diseases from the perspective of the receptor. The thesis of the participation of an active receptor in the formation of a high or, on the contrary, low tissue sensitivity to hormones is the basis of this trend.

The concentration and the properties of receptor proteins which specifically bind hormones have been investigated as a comparatively simple and reliably valuable diagnostic test for revealing a number of diseases.[63]

One of the most important factors in determining the value of a biological response to a steroid hormone is the concentration of the hormone-receptor complex which is present in the nuclei. It depends on two parameters: concentration of the hormone and receptor cellular concentration.

The absence or a considerable reduction in the content of cytoplasmic androgen receptors leads to the loss of hormone interaction with the nucleic structural components and may be attributed to the initial manifestations of the biochemical mechanisms of testicular feminization seen in males and confirmed by experiments on animals. The content of cytoplasmic androgen receptors is regulated by the level of androgens and reduction in the content of androgen receptors in seminal vesicles, prostate, and skeletal muscles after castration and may serve as one of the manifestations of such an intracellular control. A gradual reduction in cytoplasmic androgen receptor concentration leads to an actual disappearance of nuclear androgen receptors 6 to 7 days after castration.[64] It should be taken into consideration that a high lability of androgen receptors and their high activity makes it difficult to obtain reliable, repeated results and hence results in contradictory data.

Testicular feminization is an example that shows the importance of having normal levels of androgen receptors in sex organs. There is a hereditary disease linked with the X-chromosome and manifested in the form of male pseudohermaphroditism that occurs in humans and animals. It often happens that this disease does not disturb the synthesis of testosterone and its conversion to dihydrotestosterone. Some experiments on mice with Tfm (complete feminization) have allowed the determination of the essential changes in the receptor of testosterone and dihydrotestosterone in a number of androgen-dependent tissues. Results show that in these tissues, androgen binding by receptors was absent or constituted only a small part of the binding observed in analogous tissues of healthy animals. It is characteristic that the binding ability of cytoplasmic androgen receptors, as well as the ability of hormone-receptor complexes to be translocated to the nucleus, practically do not change. The basic properties of androgen receptors in mice and healthy Tfm animals do not have essential differences. However, the amount of androgen receptor in Tfm animals is considerably smaller and in a number of tissues is completely absent. Thus for this disease, the synthesis of receptors is disturbed and it is associated with the inhibition of androgen-receptor gene expression in the nuclei of sex system cells.[65]

The methods of determining steroid hormone receptors have been practiced on a large scale by revealing and treating diverse tumors in humans. The therapeutics of breast cancer has achieved the greatest development. The determination of estrogen receptors is used here as a rather informative test.[66] It turns out that cytoplasmic and nuclear estrogen receptors from cancer tissue (according to their physical-chemical properties) do not differ from normal tissue. However the amount of estrogen receptors in malignant tumors is considerably higher than in normal tissues. The determination of estrogen receptors by the therapeutics of breast cancer has allowed a considerable increase in the efficiency of conservative treatment.[67] Prostate adenoma also pertains to hormone-feeding tumors. Testosterone is able to stimulate the reproduction of tumor cells while estrogen exerts an opposing action and impedes this process. Androgen receptors, specifically binding 5α-dihydrotestosterone and testosterone, were revealed in cytosol, nuclei of human prostate cells and various tumors. However, the concentration of these receptors is rather low and their high lability creates serious methodological difficulties for practical use in clinical endocrinology. Experiments studying the reception of steroid hormones in liver, where the basic metabolic processes associated with hormone biotransformation are carried out, are of certain significance for raising the effectiveness of various hormones.

By studying the effect of AAS in human organisms, it should be taken into account that this group of steroids may cause both positive and negative alterations in metabolism. As a rule, principal attention is paid to positive alterations stipulated by an AAS anabolic effect. As for the possibility of separate links of intracellular metabolic disturbances, which are the basis of developing a negative phenomenon leading to some pathological alterations in a number of organs and tissues, they are very seldom marked. AAS are known to actively participate in the regulation of intracellular metabolism and are able to exert an influence on the function of many organs. The manifestation of the effects of AAS (positive or negative) depends on the type of AAS, the hormone dosage, the method of introduction into the organism, and the duration of hormone application. It is impossible to ignore the fact that besides clinical medicine, AAS have been used on a large scale in the field of amateur and professional sports as one of the possible ways of increasing human physical work capacity.[1,6,17] By the decision of the Medical Commission of the International Olympic Committee, AAS were attributed to doping and their application by athletes was prohibited. To uphold this decision, at all the big competitions representatives of the Medical Commission of the IOC and international federations in a variety of sports started carrying out regular doping control of athletes. There appeared the necessity to carry out special investigations to ascertain positive and negative effects of AAS application in a healthy man during systematic physical exercise.

The investigations carried out on six athletes practicing weight-lifting and taking 5 to 10 mg/day of methandrostenolone during 12 weeks with addition of special protein-mineral products did not give convincing proof of the efficiency of AAS on the development of special physical qualities.[68] The authors investigated 24 various biochemical indices of blood and skeletal muscles which made it possible to obtain a sufficiently complete notion about the state of metabolism in the subjects before AAS intake, as well as 4 and 12 weeks after the daily use of hormones. The values of separate indices of energy, protein, and lipid metabolism, as well as the activity of aminotransferase, alkali phosphatase and lactate dehydrogenase, fluctuated within the limits of the values taken as a standard for healthy men. Thus, for 12 weeks of the experiment, no decline was observed in the state of health in subjects who had taken such dosages of AAS. The use of nandrolone-decanoate in dosages of 50 mg (5 times every other day) reduced the content of general thyroxine and thyroxine-binding capability of blood in the athletes. Under these conditions, an increase in the level of free thyroxine and hypophysis thyrotropic hormone was marked.[69]

As Lamb[70] states, some experimental investigations on animals and some clinical observations on humans suppose the notion that therapeutic doses of AAS may exert a positive effect on increase in body weight and muscular mass as well as the formation of erythrocytes. However, this is only seen in organisms with low-functioning sex glands.[71] Comparison of a series of works in which AAS was used for improving physical work capacity and increasing body weight showed no convincing evidence that these hormones had a positive influence.[72-74] On the contrary, a prolonged intake of large doses of AAS leads to a disturbance in liver function and is reflected in the activity of the sex glands. In the end it exerts a negative influence on the state of human health.[75-82]

The possibility of male sex hormones participating in the metabolic regulation of muscular adaptation to physical activity is perhaps one of the most disputable problems in current endocrinology. In our opinion this has formed a paradoxical situation. On the one hand, we have studied in depth the effect of physical exercise on various functional systems in an organism. This consists of increasing the possibility of substrate mobilization and activation of the mechanisms of energy production as well as stimulation of anabolic processes during rehabilitation after physical exercise.[83-85] On the other hand, we have accumulated a large experimental database indicating the participation of androgens in the regulation of energy and protein metabolism. Their common anabolic effects include the action of androgens on the biochemical processes in skeletal muscle.[86-89] However, up to now the basic molecular-biological mechanisms by which these hormones may influence the development of the organism's adaptation to systematic physical exercise have not been discovered.

Conditionally, this problem may be divided into two aspects having independent significance. The first consists of studying the influence of muscular activity on the level of androgens in the blood and the velocity of their synthesis, metabolism, and excretion. The second aspect consists of investigating the influence of single and systematic physical exercise on the realization of the effect of androgens at a cellular level in target organs.

Let us consider the influence of physical exercise on the level of androgens in blood. The concentration of the basic hormone from the group of androgens-testosterone is known to make up 0.3 to 10 mg/ml of serum. Therefore, the study of the influence of physical exercise on the level of this hormone became possible only in the last 10 to 15 years with the advent of radioimmunoanalysis. It should be immediately noted that a generalized analysis of the results obtained at present represents a certain difficulty. It is due to the fact that the experiments were carried out on diverse subjects using physical exercises which differed according to their trend, intensity and duration.

The investigations carried out in detail on athletes using a wide range of physical exercises established[90,91] that the level of testosterone and other andro-gen-androstenediols increased during intensive muscular activity. The greatest level was seen during anaerobic physical exercise for about an hour. Analogous results were obtained in an experiment on animals in our department.[92] The type of exercise we used was repeated swimming bouts of 1 minute with rest intervals for 1.5 minutes. With a weight equaling 13 to 19% of body weight, the total duration of the work bout was 20 to 60 minutes depending on the animal's ability. It was established that the muscular activity was accompanied by an increase in the concentration of testosterone in blood by 30 to 50%. A more pronounced increase in the hormone level was observed in the animals that adapted to the physical loads.

Investigations in which the results show a rise in androgen content in male and female blood after performing physical exercise associated with weight lifting are worthy of note.[93,94] Immediately after cessation of exercise, a sharper rise in the concentration of testosterone in blood was found in men in comparison to women. Thirty minutes after exercise a lowering of testosterone content to the level of rest was observed. The same changes were marked in the content of androstenediol, but in this case the rise in steroid concentration in both men and women occurred immediately after exercise and then gradually was reduced. Thirty minutes after exercise the content of androstenediol was back to the level of rest and 2 hours later it was considerably lower than the initial values.[93] After performing strength physical exercises the content of testosterone in blood in women was low and, as a result, a pronounced effect on skeletal muscle hypertro-phy was absent.[95—98] On the other hand, it should be taken into account that by performing strength type of physical exercises, there is a reduction in blood plasma volume and in the index of hematocrit. In a number of works, a pronounced increase in testosterone content in the blood of subjects after performing physical exercises of a cyclic character (running, cycling, rowing) was seen.[100,101] For many years a group of Finnish investigators, under Prof. Adlercreutz, systematically investigated the influence of different types and intensities of physical loads on the content of some hormones in blood.[97,100,101] These works established that physical exercises lead to changes in the concen-trations of a number of hormones in the blood. Under these conditions, the application of AAS (methandienone) causes a decrease in the content of testos-terone and luteinizing and follicle stimulating hormones in blood.[102]

The experiments carried out in our laboratory established that intensive physical exercise caused essential changes in testosterone concentration in blood during muscular activity and immediately postexercise. Four hours after com-pleting muscular activity, the content of testosterone in the blood of animals increased 2.0 to 2.5 times. By injecting 19-nortestosterone into animals prior to physical exercise, changes in testosterone content in blood were the same. On the other hand, there are also contrary data. Animals running on a treadmill for 1 to 3 hours showed a reduction in testosterone concentration in blood immediately after physical exercise and an hour postexercise.[103] A decrease in the content of progesterone, androstenediol, and testosterone in testicles of animals performing physical exercises was also noted. A possible explanation for such changes in testosterone content is the inhibition of its synthesis in testicles during physical exercise. Evidence for this explanation is seen in the reduction in the concentration of this hormone in blood.

By examining the data stated above, two questions arise. First is which molecular mechanisms ensure the rise of testosterone concentration during the performance of intensive physical exercise? Secondly, and in our opinion more essential, is what functional significance may the increased hormone level have? It should be admitted that at present it is not possible to answer these questions in a reasonable way. We could only notice that the rise in testosterone concentration is apparently not due to an increase in its synthesis under the influence of luteinizing hormone.[100,102]

It is more difficult to raise a question concerning a functional role for the increase in the hormone concentration with a pronounced anabolic effect during physical exercise, which is the period when the processes of catabolism are activated. Perhaps the fact noted above is the consequence of a nonspecific reaction of the system of production and androgen metabolism under the influence of a stress character. The androgens acquire an essential functional significance as regulators of biopolymerase synthesis at a remote period of rehabilitation after physical exercise. It was shown that after completing the muscular activity phase, alterations in the testosterone level were observed.[92] The concentration of testosterone decreased to low values during the first 1.5 to 2.0 hours of rest, and then a gradual rise of hormone level up to the 6th to 7th hour of the rest period was observed. The range of testosterone concentration in blood increased with the rise in the physical fitness of the animal. It may be also noted that a reduction in the testosterone and androstenediol levels during the period of rest after physical exercise was shown in experiments on athletes as well.[89] Recovery, however, to initial concentrations occurred later, sometimes 24 to 48 hours.

On the grounds of the results of the investigations discussed, one can hypothesize that systematic physical exercise can cause considerable hormonal alterations in an organism. Evidence for this is seen by changes in the ratio of sex hormones to the appearance of hyperandrogenemia symptoms. With the factors accompanying this phenomenon, an increase in testicular activity may first be seen, then a reduction in blood volume, and last, intensification of the peripheral mechanism of the formation of androgens. Some possible pathways of regulation of the level of androgens in blood are given in Figure 23.

It should be noted that the ability of metabolites, which are formed during the performance of physical exercise, to exert a direct effect on hormone-determining organs or exert a regulatory action through the hypothalamic-pituitary system is of great significance although it practically remains unstudied. The elucidation of these questions will allow a more detailed study of the biochemical processes associated with androgen participation in the regulation of intracellular metabolism both during and after physical exercise.

It is necessary to mention one more sphere of wide AAS application: meat

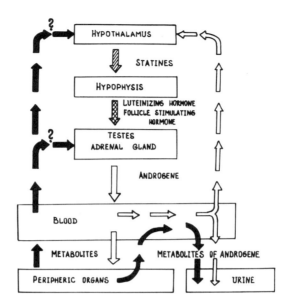

FIGURE 23.   Possible ways of the regulation of androgen level in blood.[89]

production. The use of synthetic hormones for raising productivity in animal husbandry originated in 1938 when the synthesis of estrogen derivatives (diethylstilbestrol) was accomplished. In later years this hormone was used widely in cattle breeding in a number of countries up to the middle 70s, when there appeared some reports about essential disturbances in human health after eating meat products that contained diethylstilbestrol. Some countries, such as Italy, made a decision to prohibit the use of anabolic agents for raising productivity in animal husbandry. Some intensive investigations by a number of pharmaceutical firms led to the synthesis of new hormones of various nature. Among them were the anabolic steroid trenbolone-acetate, a vegetable hormone of nonsteroid origin, zeranol, and several progestin derivatives. These are hormones that have been used on a large scale in cattle breeding as well as in research work.[105,106] Only recently have radioimmunoassay techniques been developed that can trace these hormones in animal tissue and biological liquids.[106,107] This has allowed the discovery of the principal metabolic pathways of trenbolone-acetate and zeranol in animal organisms[108-110] as well as a way to choose convenient forms for introducing hormones into an organism and determining the time and forms of their excretion.

Of the three methods of AAS introduction which are commonly used in cattle breeding (oral, injection and implantation), implantation is the most popular. At present, most anabolic agents are introduced into animals in the form of implants. It has been established that the best results concerning animals growth weight were obtained just after implantation of hormone mixtures.[111-115] The use of anabolic agents, including AAS, on the grounds of food ration balanced by basic nutrition factors leads to a certain growth of body mass.[116,117] In different investigations this value fluctuates within sufficiently large limits, but as a rule, such growth weight due to AAS application can make up 10 to 20%.[118-120] A wide use of AAS in cattle breeding led to the need to create special recommendations to determine the conditions of hormone usage (doses, dates, forms of introduction, animal age, etc.). In addition, there appeared a need to determine ways to control AAS application in different countries. Suffice it to note that in England 25 to 30% of total meat production is obtained by using anabolic agents. The working group of WHO experts considered the list of anabolic agents used in cattle breeding and recommended the use of trenbolone-acetate and zeranol. At the same time, since July 1982, the use of diethylstilbestrol and other stilbene derivatives as a means of stimulating growth in cattle breeding has been prohibited in all countries.[121,122]

The application of anabolic agents including AAS in cattle breeding is based on a thorough study of the metabolism of these substances in various tissues of animals which are used for meat production. As the recommendations for farmers state, the level of synthetic hormones introduced into an organism is not to exceed that of endogenic hormones (androgens and estrogens). During slaughtering, the anabolic agents and their metabolites must be absent in animal tissues. The experience of cattle breeding in England shows that the production of meat using AAS gives a certain economic effect, and by following the recommendations of the working group of WHO experts, the consumption of such meat is quite safe for the population. At the same time, it is necessary to carry out a systematic control for AAS application during fattening. For this reason, up-to-date physical-chemical methods may be used. They allow the determination of AAS and their metabolites in human and animal tissues and biological liquids.

REFERENCES

1. Johnson L. C. and O'Shea, J. P., Anabolic steroids: effects on strength development, *Science,* 164, 957, 1969.
2. Pongratz, D. and Mittlebach, F., Influence of anabolic steroids on normal and denervated skeletal muscle, *Excer. Med. Endocrinol.,* 23, 68, 1969.
3. O'Shea, J. and Winker, W., Biochemical and physical effects of an anabolic steroid in competitive swimmers and weight lifters, *Nutr. Rep. Int.,* 2, 351, 1970.
4. O'Shea, J. P., The effects of an anabolic steroid on dynamic strength levels of weight lifters, *Nutr. Rep. Int.,* 4, 363, 1971.
5. Casner, S. W., Early, R. C., and Carlson, B. R., Anabolic steroid effects on body composition in normal young men, *J. Sports Med. Phys. Fit.,* 11, 98, 1971.

6. **Wimnay, M. and Mya-Tu, M.,** The effects of anabolic steroids on physical fitness, *J. Sport. Med. Phys. Fit.,* 15, 266, 1975.

7. **Hervey, G. R., Knibbs, A. V., Burkinshow, L., Morgan, D. B., Jones, P. R. M., and Chetfle, D. A.,** Effects of methandienone on the performance and body compositions of men undergoing athletic training, *Clin. Sci.,* 60, 457, 1981.

8. **Bowes, R. W. and Rearden, J. R.,** Effects of methandrostenolone (dianabol) on strength development and aerobic capacity, *Med. Sci. Sports,* 4, 54, 1972.

9. **Santidrian, S.,** Anabolic action of dianabol (17α-methyl-17β-hydroxyandrostan-1,4 dien-3-one) on the nitrogen balance and skeletal muscle composition of rats fed on field bean (*Vica faba* L), *Horm. Metabol. Res.,* 13, 407, 1981.

10. **Fowler, W. M., Gardner, G. W., and Egstrom, G. H.,** Effects of an anabolic steroid on physical performance of young men, *J. Appl. Physiol.,* 20, 1038, 1965.

11. **Stromme, S. B., Meen, J. D., and Aakvaac, A.,** Effects of an androgenic-anabolic steroid on strength development and plasma testosterone levels in normal males, *Med. Sci. Sports,* 6, 203, 1974.

12. **Crist, D. M., Stackpole, P. J., and Peaks, G. T.,** Effect of androgenic-anabolic steroid on neuromuscular power and body composition, *J. Appl. Physiol.,* 54, 366, 1983.

13. **Max, S. R. and Toop, J.,** Androgens enhance in vivo 2-deoxyglucose uptake by rat striated muscle, *Endocrinology,* 113, 119, 1983.

14. **Landon, J., Wynn, V., and Samols, E.,** The effect of anabolic steroids in blood sugar and plasma insulin levels in man, *Metabolism,* 12, 924, 1963.

15. **Szikantia, S. G.,** Effect of a C17-alkylated steroid methandrostenolone on plasma lipids of normal subjects, *Am. J. Med. Sci.,* 254, 201, 1967.

16. **Gribbin, H. R. and Flavell Matts, S. G.,** Mode of action and use of anabolic steroids, *Br. J. Clin. Pract.,* 30, 3, 1976.

17. **Wright, J. E.,** *Anabolic Steroids and Sports,* Sport Science Consultants, Natick, MA, 1978.

18. **Zarubina, N. A.,** Anabolic steroids, their basic properties and clinical application, *Sov. Med.,* 5, 83, 1982.

19. **Goldstein, J. L. and Brown, M. S.,** Lipoprotein receptors, cholesterol metabolism and atherosclerosis, *Arch. Pathol.,* 99, 181, 1975.

20. **Goldstein, J. L. and Brown, M. S.,** Atherosclerosis: the low-density lipoprotein receptor hypothesis, *Metabolism,* 26, 1257, 1977.

21. **Goldstein, J. L. and Brown, M. S.,** The low-density lipoprotein pathway and its relation to atherosclerosis, *Annu. Rev. Biochem.,* 46, 897, 1977.

22. **Taggart, H. M. and Appelbaum-Bowden, D.,** Reduction in high density lipoproteins by anabolic steroid (stanozolol) therapy for postmenopausal osteoporosis, *Metab. Clin. Exp.,* 31, 1147, 1982.

23. **Haffner, S. M., Kushwaha, R. S., and Foster, D. H.,** The metabolic mechanism of reduced high density lipoproteins during anabolic steroid therapy, *Metab. Clin. Exp.,* 32, 413, 1983.

24. **Korge, P. and Rooson, S.,** The importance of adrenal gland in the improved adaptation of trained animals to physical exertion, *Endocrinology,* 64, 232, 1975.

25. **Viru, A. A.,** The functions of adrenal cortex by muscular activities, *Medicine,* Moscow, 1977.

26. **Hervey, G. R. and Hutchimson, J.,** Anabolic effects of methandienone in men undergoing athletic training, *Lancet,* p. 699, October 2, 1976.

27. **Vermeulen, A.,** Influence of anabolic steroids on secretion and metabolism of cortisol, in *Structure and Metabolism of Corticosteroids,* Pasqualini, J. R. and Jayle, M. F., Eds., Academic Press, New York, 1964, 109.

28. **Johnsen, S. G.,** Maintenance of spermatogenesis induced by HMG treatment by means of continuous HGC treatment in hypogonadotrophic men, *Acta Endocrinol.,* 89, 763, 1978.

29. **Letschinsky, L. A. and Shenkareva, S. A.,** On using steroid and nonsteroid anabolics by heart ischemia, *Clin. Med.,* N4, 38, 1976.

30. **Letschinsky, L. A., Bryskina, G. S., and Demina, L. A.,** The experience on using combined

pharmacotherapeutics by immune depressanters and anabolic steroids by a series of inflammatory and dystrophic processes in clinic of internal diseases, *Ther. Arch.*, N11, 67, 1977.

31. **Bei, P. I.**, Nerabol effect on contractile capability of myocardia, *Clin. Med.*, 50, 69, 1972.

32. **Chimenko, L. P.**, Dynamics of clinico-biochemical indices in postinfarction cardiosclerosis sick persons with stenocardia syndrome by treatment with anabolic steroids, *Clin. Med.*, 59, 42, 1981.

33. **Deineko, N. F., Shustval, N. F., and Ichnenko, R. I.**, Treatment of ulcer with anabolic hormones, *Clin. Med.*, 51, 57, 1973.

34. **Zaporozhts, V. K.**, The application of anabolic steroids by operative treatment of sick persons with stenosed stomach and duodenal ulcer, *Clin. Surg.*, N8, 82, 1978.

35. **Bodnja, I. A.**, Anabolic hormones as a means of electrolytic exchange by chronic enterocolitis in children, *Pediatrics*, N7, 26, 1973.

36. **Yatschenko, B. M., Berezatsky, A. V., and Babinskaya, I. P.**, Anabolic steroids in complex treatment of sick persons with pulmonary tuberculosis at elderly and old ages, *Probl. Tuberc.*, N1, 26, 1980.

37. **Silvestrov, V. P. and Einer, E. A.**, Effect of anabolic steroid Anadur on humoral immunity and "sharp-phase" proteins by acute pneumonia, *Pharm. Toxicol.*, 45, 100, 1982.

38. **Taxanori, N., Yamagishi, M., and Uchino, H.**, Effect of various androgens on hematopoiesis, *Acta Haematol. Jpn.*, 44, 812, 1981.

39. **Fairhead, S. M., Chipping, P. M., and Gorsonsmith, E. C.**, Treatment of aplastic anemia with antilymphocyte globulin, *Br. J. Haematol.*, 55, 7, 1983.

40. **Chang, J. C., Slutzker, B., and Lindsay, N.**, Case report, remission of pure red cell aplasia following oxymetholone therapy, *Am. J. Med. Sci.*, 275, 345, 1978.

41. **Lockner, D.**, Treatment of refractory anemias with methenolone, *Acta Med. Scand.*, 205, 97, 1979.

42. **Hast, R., Engstedt, L., and Jameson, S.**, Oxymetholone treatment in myelofibrosis, *Blut*, 37, 19, 1978.

43. **Branda, R. F., Amsden, T. W., and Jacob, H. S.**, Randomized study of nandrolone therapy for anemias due to bone marrow failure, *Arch. Intern. Med.*, 137, 65, 1977.

44. **Rosse, W. F., Logue, G. L., and Silberman, H. R.**, The effect of synthetic androgens in hereditary angioneurotic edema, *Trans. Assoc. Am. Phys.*, 89, 122, 1976.

45. **Gould, D. J., Cunliffe, W. J., and Smiddy, E. G.**, Anabolic steroids in hereditary angioedema, *Lancet*, 1, 770, 1978.

46. **Barbosa, J., Seal, U. S., and Doe, R. P.**, Effect of anabolic steroids on haptoglobin, orosomucoid, plasminogen, fibrinogen, transferrin, ceruloplasmin, α-antitrypsin, β-glucuronidase and total serum proteins, *J. Clin. Endocrinol.*, 33, 388, 1971.

47. **Carl-Bertil, L. and Rannevick, G.**, A comparison of plasma protein changes induced by danazol, pregnancy and estrogens, *J. Clin. Endocrinol. Metabol.*, 49, 719, 1979.

48. **Ochotsky, V. P., Dubrov, E. Ya., and Gorianova, M. G.**, Clinical experience in using thyrocalcitonin and anabolic steroids in sick persons with senile fractures of thigh-bone, *Sov. Med.*, N3, 18, 1975.

49. **Michelson, C. B., Askanazi, J., Kinney, J. H., and Gump, F. E.**, Effect of an anabolic steroid on nitrogen balance and amino acid patterns after total hip replacement, *J. Trauma*, 22, 410, 1982.

50. **Alastar, Y. G., Macfie, J., and Hill, G. L.**, The effect of an anabolic steroid on body composition in patients receiving intravenous nutrition, *Aust. N.Z. J. Surg.*, 51, 280, 1981.

51. **Verheul, H., Stimson, W. H., den Hollander, F. C., and Scheeurs, A.**, The effects of nandrolone, testosterone and their decanoate esters on neurine lupus, *Clin. Exp. Immunol.*, 44, 11, 1981.

52. **Bislama, J. W., Duursma, S. A., Bosch, R., and Huber, O.**, Lack of influence of the anabolic steroid nandrolone decanoate on boral metabolism, *Acta Endocrinol.*, 101, 140, 1982.

53. **Hazelton, R. A., Mecruden, A. B., Sturrock, R. D., and Stimson, W. H.**, Hormonal

manipulation of the immune response in systemic lupus erythematosus: a drug trial of an anabolic steroid, 19-nortestosterone, *Ann. Rheum. Dis.,* 42, 155, 1983.

54. **Harkness, R. A., Kilshaw, B. H., and Hobson, B. M.,** Effect of large doses of anabolic steroids, *Br. J. Sports Med.,* 9, 70, 1975.

55. **Goldfarb, S.,** Sex hormones and hepatic neoplasma, *Cancer Res.,* 36, 2584, 1976.

56. **Spiers, A. S., Devita, S. F., and Allar, M. J.,** Beneficial effects of an anabolic steroid during cytotoxic chemotherapy for metastatic cancer, *J. Med.,* 12, 433, 1981.

57. **Turani, H., Levi, J., Zevin, D., and Kessler, E.,** Hepatic lesions in patients on anabolic androgenic therapy, *JSR, J. Med. Sci.,* 19, 332, 1983.

58. **Zbytneiwski, Z., Kancler, A. Z., and Boaryd, B.,** Influence of aspirin and/or anabolic steroid (nandrolone decanoate) on experimental metastasis formation, *Arch. Immunol. Ther. Exp.,* 29, 697, 1981.

59. **Fannuti, F., Gaggi, R., and Murari-Colalongi, P.,** The anabolic and androgenic-antiandrogenic activity of different dose levels of oxyprogesterone acetate in rats, *Oncology,* 38, 307, 1981.

60. **Mochizuki, Y., Sawada, N., and Furukawa, K.,** Effect of bolandiol dipropionate (Anabiol) anabolic hormone on diethyl nitrosamine-induced hepatocarcinogenesis in rats, *Gann,* 72, 969, 1981.

61. **Bagheri, S. A. and Boyer, J. L.,** Peliosis hepatis associated with androgenic-anabolic steroid, *Ther. Ann. Intern. Med.,* 81, 610, 1974.

62. **Wilson, J. D. and Griffin, E.,** The use and misuse of androgens, *Metabolism,* 29, 1278, 1980.

63. **Danforth, D. N., Tamarkin, L., and Lippman, M. E.,** Melatonin increases oestrogen receptors binding activity of human breast cancer cell, *Nature,* 305, 323, 1983.

64. **Weinberger, M. J. and Veneziale, C. M.,** Nuclear acceptor sites for androgen-receptor complexes in seminal-vesicle epithelium, *Biochem. J.,* 192, 41, 1980.

65. **Mainwaring, W. J. P.,** *The Mechanism of Action of Androgens,* Springer-Verlag, New York, 1977.

66. **Seibert, K. and Lippman, M. E.,** Hormone receptor. Assays in breast cancer, *J. Clin. Immunoassay,* 6, 5, 1983.

67. **Syne, J. S. and Panko, W. B.,** New techniques for the measurement of estrogen receptor in human breast cancer, *J. Clin. Immunoassay,* 6, 17 (Suppl.) 1983.

68. **Edgerton, V. R., Garhammer, J. J., Simpson, D. R., and Campion, D. S.,** Case studies of competitive weight lifters taking anabolic steroids, in *Medicine and Sports,* Leningrad, 1979, 133.

69. **Smirnova, L. K., Semenov, V. A., Seifulla, R. D., Kuterove, O. A., and Mansvetova, E. V.,** Effect of retabolil on functional activity of thyroid hormones in athletes, *Pharmacol. Toxicol. (USSR),* 46, 79, 1983.

70. **Lamb, D. R.,** Anabolic-androgenic steroids and athletic performance, in *Medicine and Sports,* Leningrad, 1979, 108.

71. **Lamb, D. R.,** Anabolic steroids in athletics: how well do they work and how dangerous are they?, *Am. J. Sports Med.,* 12, 31, 1984.

72. **Ryan, A. J.,** Anabolic steroids are fool's gold, *Fed. Proc.,* 40, 2682, 1981.

73. American College of Sports Medicine. Position statement on the use and abuse of anabolic-androgenic steroids in sports, *Med. Sci. Sports,* 9, xi-xiii, 1977.

74. **Max, S. R. and Rance, N. E.,** No effect of sex steroids on compensatory muscle hypertrophy, *J. Appl. Physiol.,* 56, 1989, 1984.

75. **Begheri, S. A. and Boyer, J. L.,** Peliosis hepatitis associated with androgenic-anabolic steroid therapy, *Ann. Int. Med.,* 81, 610, 1974.

76. **Falk, H., Thomas, L. B., Popper, H., and Isaak, K. G.,** Hepatic angiosarcoma associated with androgenic-anabolic steroids, *Lancet,* 1, 1120, 1979.

77. **Guy, J. T. and Auslander, M. O.,** Androgenic steroids and hepatocellular carcinoma, *Lancet,* 1, 148, 1975.

78. **Henderson, J. T., Richmond, J., and Sumerling, M. D.,** Androgenic-anabolic steroid therapy and hepatocellular carcinoma, *Lancet,* 1, 934, 1972.
79. **Holms, P. K.,** Effect of an anabolic steroid (methandienone) on spermatogenesis, *Contraception,* 15, 151, 1979.
80. **Mc Donald, E. C. and Speicher, C. E.,** Peliosis hepatitis associated with administration of oxymetholone, *J. Am. Med. Assoc.,* 240, 243, 1978.
81. **Noble, R. L.,** Androgen use by athletes: a possible cancer risk, *Can. Med. Assoc. J.,* 130, 549, 1984.
82. **Johnson, D. A.,** Use of anabolic steroids by athletes, *JAMA,* 251, 1430, 1984.
83. **Yakovlev, N. N.,** Biochemistry of sports, *Phys. Cult. Sports,* Moscow, 1974.
84. **Rogozkin, V. A.,** Metabolic effect of anabolic steroid on skeletal muscle, *Med. Sci. Sports,* 11, 160, 1979.
85. **Viru, A. A. and Korge, P. K.,** Hormones and efficiency, *Phys. Cult. Sports,* Moscow, 1983.
86. **Lamb, D.,** Androgens and exercise, *Med. Sci. Sports,* 7, 1, 1975.
87. **Rogozkin, V. A.,** Anabolic steroid metabolism in skeletal muscle, *J. Steroid Biochem.,* 11, 923, 1979.
88. **Viru, A. A. and Korge, P. K.,** Role of anabolic steroid in the hormonal regulation of skeletal muscle adaptation, *J. Steroid Biochem.,* 11, 931, 1979.
89. **Rogozkin, V. A. and Feldkoren, B. I.,** Androgens and adaptation of the organism to physical exercises, in *Muscular Activity and Hormones,* Leningrad, 1982, 6.
90. **Kuoppsalmi, K., Näveri, H., Harkönen, M., and Adlercreutz, H.,** Plasma cortisol, androstendione, testosterone and luteinizing hormone in running exercises of different intensities, *Scand. J. Clin. Lab. Invest.,* 40, 403, 1980.
91. **Langer, H., Buhl, H., Neumann, G., and Sattler, R.,** *Med. Sport,* 9, 287, 1981.
92. **Kotsegub, T. P. and Feldcoren, B. I.,** Effect of physical exercises on the content of testosterone in blood in trained rats, in *Endocrine Mechanisms of Regulation of the Adaptation to Muscular Activities, Tartu,* X, 138, 1980.
93. **Weiss, L. W., Gureton, K. J., and Thompson, F. N.,** Comparison of serum testosterone and androgendione responses to weight lifting in men and women, *Eur. J. Appl. Physiol.,* 50, 413, 1983.
94. **Fahey, T., Rolph, R., Mongmee, P., Nagel, J., and Mortora, S.,** Serum testosterone, body composition and strength of young adults, *Med. Sci. Sports,* 8, 31, 1976.
95. **Brown, C. and Wilmore, J.,** The effects of maximal resistance training on the strength and body composition of women athletes, *Med. Sci. Sports,* 6, 174, 1974.
96. **Wilmore, J.,** Alterations in strength, body composition and anthropometric measurements consequent to a 10-week weight training program, *Med. Sci. Sports,* 6, 133, 1974.
97. **Kuoppasalmi, K., Näveri, H., Rehunen, S., Harkönen, M., and Adlercreuz, H.,** Effect of strenuous anaerobic running exercise on plasma growth hormone, cortisol, luteinizing hormone, testosterone, androstendione, estrone and estradiol, *J. Steroid Biochem.,* 7, 823, 1976.
98. **Hetrick, G. and Wilmore, J.,** Androgen levels and muscle hypertrophy during an eight week weight training program for men/women, *Med. Sci. Sports Exerc.,* 11, 102, 1979.
99. **Mc Connel, T. R. and Sinning, W. E.,** Exercise and temperature effects on human sperm production and testosterone levels, *Med. Sci. Sports Exerc.,* 16, 51, 1984.
100. **Adlercreutz, H.,** Physical activity and hormones, *Adv. Cardiol.,* 18, 144, 1976.
101. **Kuoppasolmi, K.,** Plasma testosterone and sex-hormone-binding globulin in physical exercise, *Scand. J. Clin. Lab. Invest.,* 40, 411, 1980.
102. **Holma, P. and Adlercreutz, H.,** Effect of an anabolic steroid (methandienone) on plasma LH, ESH, testosterone and on the response to intravenous administration of LRH, *Acta Endocrinol.,* 83, 856, 1976.
103. **Harkönen, M., Juoppasalmi, K., Näveri, H., and Karonen, S. L.,** Regulation of plasma androgens in muscular exercise, *J. Clin. Chem. Clin. Biochem.,* 19, 689, 1981.

104. **Wise, D. R. and Ranaweera, K. N.,** Effect of trienbolone acetate and other anabolic agents in growth of turkeys, *Br. Poult. Sci.,* 22, 93, 1981.
105. **Sinett-Smith, P. A., Dumelow, N. W., and Buttery, P. J.,** Effect of trenbolone acetate and zeranol on protein metabolism in male castrated and female lambs, *Br. J. Nutr.,* 50, 225, 1983.
106. **Dixon, S. N.,** Radioimmunoassay of the anabolic agent zeranol, *J. Vet. Pharm. Ther.,* 3, 177, 1980.
107. **Dixon, S. N. and Russell, K. L.,** Radioimmunoassay of the anabolic agent zeranol, *J. Vet. Pharm. Ther.,* 6, 173, 1983.
108. **Rico, A. G.,** Metabolism of endogenous and exogenous anabolic agents in cattle, *J. Anim. Sci.,* 57, 226, 1983.
109. **Migdolof, B. H., Dugger, H. A., Heider, J. G., and Coombs, R. A.,** Biotransformation of zeranol: disposition and metabolism in the female rat, rabbit, dog, monkey and man, *Xenobiotica,* 13, 209, 1983.
110. **Salmons, S.,** Myotrophic effects of anabolic steroids, *Vet. Res. Commun.,* 7, 19, 1983.
111. **Richardson, T. C., Jeacock, M. K., and Schepherd, D. A.,** The effect of implantation of anabolic steroids into suckling ruminating lambs on the metabolism of alanine in livers perfused in the presence and absence of volatile fatty acids, *J. Agric. Sci.,* 99, 391, 1982.
112. **Harrison, L. P., Heitzman, R. J., and Sanson, B. F.,** The absorption of anabolic agents from pellets implanted at the base of the ear in sheep, *J. Vet. Pharm. Ther.,* 6, 293, 1983.
113. **Harisson, R. D.,** Effects on the anabolic steroid trenbolone acetate implanted alone or in combination with estradiol-17 on liver cell ultrastructure in steers, *Res. Vet. Sci.,* 36, 34, 1983.
114. **O'Lambna, M.,** Effect of repeated implantation with anabolic agents on growth rate, carcass weight, testicular size and behaviour of bulls, *Vet. Res.,* 113, 531, 1983.
115. **Snow, D. H., Munro, C. D., Nimmo, M. A.,** Effects of nandrolone phenylpropionate in the horse, *Equine Vet. J.,* 14, 219, 1982.
116. **Metcalf, W., Blumberg, H., and Roach, J.,** A quantitative expression for nitrogen retention with anabolic steroids. IV. Oxandrolone *Metab. Clin. Exp.,* 14, 59, 1965.
117. **Donaldson, I. A., Hart, I. C., and Heitzman, R. J.,** Growth hormone, insulin, prolactin and total thyroxine in the plasma of sheep implanted with the anabolic steroid trenbolone acetate alone or with oestradiol, *Res. Vet. Sci.,* 30, 7, 1981.
118. **Reynolds, I. P.,** Correct use of anabolic agents in ruminants, *Vet. Res.,* 107, 367, 1980.
119. **Quirke, J. F. and Sheehan, W.,** Effects of anabolic steroids on the performance of hill and low land lambs, *Ir. J. Agric. Res.,* 20, 125, 1981.
120. **Buttery, P. J. and Sinneff-Smith, P. A.,** The mode of action of anabolic agents with special reference to their effects on protein metabolism — some speculations, *Curr. Top. Vet. Med. Anim. Sci.,* 26, 211, 1984.
121. Editorial, *Lancet,* 1, 721, 1982.
122. Working Group on Health Aspects of Residues of Anabolics in Meat, ICP/FSP 002(I)(S) 8467B, World Health Organization-Regional Office for Europe, Bilthoven, The Netherlands, November 13, 1981.

Chapter 8

AAS RADIOIMMUNOASSAY

Radioimmunoassay (RIA) is one of the variants of saturation analyses in which antibodies are used as a binding substance and an antigen is used as a ligand. The RIA principle is based on antigen binding to an antibody in the presence of diverse antigen quantities. In accordance with the law of mass action, if the solution contains an antigen (Ag) and a specific antibody (Ab), a dynamic balance is established between them:

$$Ag + Ab \underset{K_2}{\overset{K_1}{\rightleftharpoons}} Ag \cdot Ab \qquad (8)$$

by which:

$$\frac{(Ag\ Ab)}{(Ag) \cdot (Ab)} = \frac{K_1}{K_2} = K \qquad (9)$$

where K_1 and K_2 are constants of direct and reverse reactions, respectively. Ag, Ab and Ag · Ab are molecular concentrations of free antigen, antibody, and the complex of antigen-antibody, while K is the constant of equilibrium which characterizes the antibody affinity for the antigen. The precise meaning of an equilibrium concentration depends on the energy of the antibody binding to antigen. The value K is a measure of the free energy change in the reaction between Ag and Ab. By a constant quantity of binding substance (antibody) and a given value K, the ratio of the binding ligand (antigen) to the free one in a state of equilibrium is in quantitative dependence on the total quantity of the ligand present.[1]

In other words, the antigen distribution between free and bound forms is in direct dependence on the total quantity of antigen present which determines its quantity. The antigens labeled by radioactive isotopes, most frequently ^{125}I or [33]H, are used for a precise determination of antigen-antibody complex. The use of radioactive ligand allows the rapid and precise measurement of ligand distribution between free and bound fractions. It is necessary to emphasize an important point which is often forgotten when describing RIA. The final distribution of ligand in free and bound fractions is determined only by the total quantity of the ligand and does not depend on the ratio of the quantities of labeled or unlabeled ligand. Both labeled and unlabeled ligand are bound to an antibody in equal proportions with no competition for binding sites on the antibody, as the reference book on the radioimmunochemical method of investigation notes.[2] RIA possesses a number of advantages over other methods of AAS determination: high sensitivity, specificity, precision, and reliability, the possibility of standardizing the procedure of analysis, and using computers for the calculations. The conditions for the application of RIA for steroid hormone determination are examined in detail in a number of monographs and reviews.[1,3-5]

Thus, to carry out RIA of AAS , it is necessary to have:

1. Labeled AAS ligands and
2. Antiserum for AAS antibodies.

Let us examine some principal conditions for obtaining labeled ligands in order to determine AAS by means of RIA.

In a perfect RIA, the radioactive labeled and unlabeled steroid must not differ in chemical or immunologic characteristics. To obtain a radioactive ligand one most often uses the isotope ^{125}I with a half-life of 56 days, ^{131}I with a shorter half-life of 8 days, ^{3}H with a half-life of 12.3 years, or seldom used ^{14}C with a half-life of 5730 years.[6] In recent years considerable success in the synthesis of deuterated labeled steroids of different classes has been achieved. Deuterium of steroid molecules has two essential advantages. Such molecules are chemically indistinguishable from unlabeled analogues. However, they can be determined by means of physical methods using nuclear magnetic resonance or a mass spectrometry. Additionally, the introduction of deuterium into the steroid molecule does not increase the toxicity of the substance.

There are two methods of preparing radioactively labeled ligands. In the first method the ligand contains an internal marker and the atom of some element, which is present in the molecule, is substituted for a radioactive isotope of the same element. For the steroid hormone and especially for AAS, ^{3}H is most frequently used instead of ^{1}H. The atoms of tritium and hydrogen are very similar to each other in size and chemical properties and the antibodies possess the same affinity for native and tritium steroids. This is a significant advantage from the point of view of obtaining reliable data, as well as for potentially standardizing RIAs in different laboratories. For the second method, an external mark in the ligand molecule is created by means of substituting one or more atoms in the structure of a low molecular substance for radioactive isotope atoms. It is then combined with the ligand by a covalent bond. The isotopes ^{125}I and ^{131}I are usually used for introducing the external mark. The ligand containing the external mark has some chemical differences from the unlabeled ligand, although according to immunological properties they are practically identical. The ligands labeled with iodine isotopes possess highly specific radioactivity. As a rule, it is one order higher than that of the tritium combination. For this reason attempts were made to introduce ^{125}I into the steroid molecule as an internal mark.[8] However, it should be noted that by using iodated steroids, there exists a considerable defect which is the result of a frequent change in the labeled ligand due to a short half-life of the radioactive iodine isotope.

In our work we used tritium-labeled AAS in positions 6 and 7 with specific radioactivity up to 50 Ki/mM. The synthesis of 19-nortestosterone-(6,7 ^{3}H), 17α-ethyl-19-nortestosterone-(6,7 ^{3}H) and 1-dehydro-17α-methyltestosterone-(6,7

[3]H) was carried out by using the catalytic hydrogenation of 6-dehydro derivatives of these steroids. AAS dehydrogenation was carried out using chloranile.[9]

For the purification of labeled ligands, various physical-chemical methods can be used. Most recently, the method of gel chromatography has been most commonly used on a large scale. In our laboratory, we have been using AAS labeled with tritium in positions 6 and 7 with radioactivity of 40 to 59 Ki/mM.[10] Periodically, once every 2 to 4 months, according to the steroid structure, it is necessary to subject them to purification in the column with Sephadex LH-20 (1 × 15 cm) in the system with a toluene-methanol solution (85:15).

Not only may the radioactive isotope serve as a marker, but other substances that can tightly bind to a ligand and may be precisely measured in very small quantities may also do the same. Some investigations have described the possibility of using a fluorescent substance for steroid determination[11,12] or some variants of enzyme immunoassay (EIA) of AAS in biological liquids.[13,14]

Obtaining antisera for AAS has some peculiarities and therefore it is advisable to examine this problem in more detail. AAS do not have high molecular weights (200 to 300 daltons), nor do they possess immunologic activity. To obtain antigenic properties it is necessary to covalently bind AAS to immunologic macromolecular protein. For this purpose bovine serum albumin (BSA), having a molecular mass of about 70,000 daltons, is usually used. A high immunogenic property, a good solubility, and a high stability for denaturation in chemical reactions of serum albumins make them useful as an immunogenic macromolecular carrier. Injecting into the animal organism (rat, rabbit, sheep) such a complex of AAS with BSA stimulates the formation of specific antibodies. To obtain the conjugated antigen AAS-BSA, one uses such covalent binding reactions that occur in water solutions at low temperature with neutral and weak alkali solution and which are not accompanied by protein denaturation. AAS interaction with BSA should not be carried out with basic functional groups of a steroid (hydroxyl, carbonyl and double bonds).

The synthesis of AAS conjugates with BSA consists of two stages. First, in order to form a covalent bond with protein it is necessary to obtain a steroid derivative which has a functional group. The most frequently used is carboxyl.[15] To obtain AAS derivatives according to a steroid molecular structure, keto or hydroxyl groups are used. In the first case, the amino acetic acid forming 3-(O-carboxymethyl) AAS oxime and its conjugate, with BSA, become part of the steroid, which, according to position 3, contains a keto group (Figure 24). The reaction is carried out in boiling ethanol.

In the second case, a carboxyl is introduced into the steroid molecule through a hydroxyl group in the course of reacting with the anhydride of double-base acids. Hemisuccinate is usually used for this purpose. Figure 25 shows the synthesis of 3-hemisuccinate methylandrostanediol. The reaction is carried out in boiling pyridine.

In some cases, to obtain AAS derivatives it is necessary to carry out the reduction of a 3-keto group to a hydroxyl group beforehand. An example of this

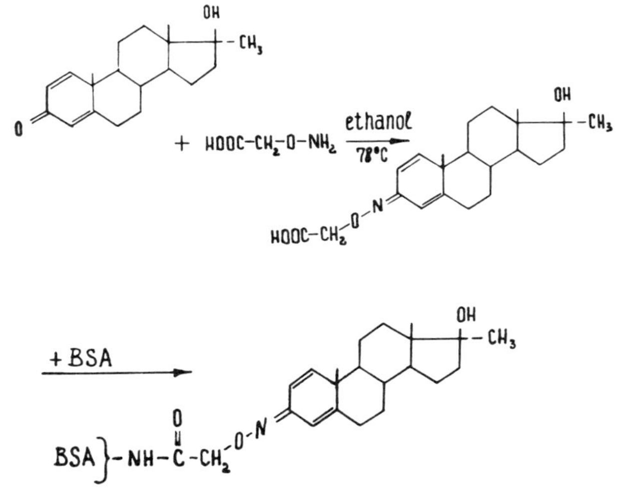

FIGURE 24. Synthesis of 3-(O-carboxymethyl)-methandrostenolone oxime and its conjugate with BSA.

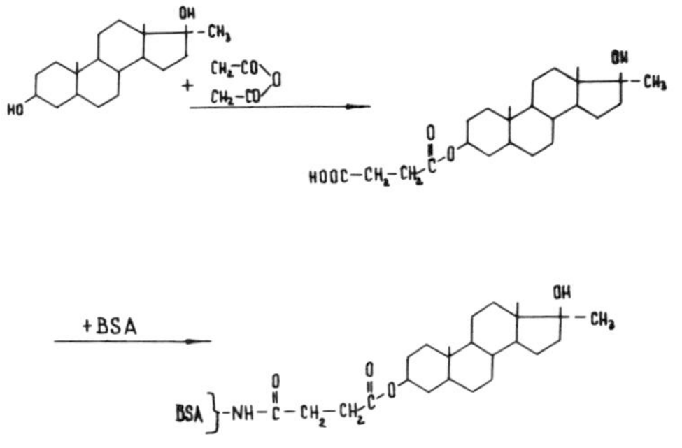

FIGURE 25. Synthesis of 3-hemisuccinate methylandrostanediol and its conjugate with BSA.

would be the way oxandrolone derivatives are obtained. AAS derivatives synthesized in this way have a carboxyl group which is used for the formation of a peptide bond with free amino groups of BSA lysine. To obtain conjugated antigens the steroid-protein carbodiimide and its derivatives are often used as a means of condensing.[16,17] In this way, the conjugated antigen AAS-BSA was synthesized for seven steroids in our laboratory.[10,18] The same AAS may be covalently bound to BSA in different ways. It is also possible to introduce new functional groups into various positions of the AAS molecule according to how the steroid combines with protein. Thus, it is possible to synthesize conjugated antigens with the same AAS which has a diverse structure with a changing character according to the position of the covalent bond between AAS and BSA.

The conjugate AAS-BSA synthesis is isolated from the reaction medium by means of either dialysis against water or gel chromatography on columns with Sephadex. To establish the presence of AAS in a conjugated antigen, it is possible to use the spectrophotometric method. By comparing UV spectra of the initial BSA and the synthesized conjugate, one can determine the number of AAS molecules bound to protein. The application of AAS as an immunogenic protein is rather preferable mainly because we know its initial structure and, in addition, the number of lysine residue has been precisely determined to be 59. Theoretically, one albumin molecule is able to bind 60 AAS molecules (59 lysine radicals and terminal NH_2). However, in practice and as a rule, one gets values equal to 20 to 30 bound AAS per one BSA molecule. This is due to a secondary structure of protein and the protection of half of the NH_2-lysine groups.[19,20] However, even with such values, the BSA conjugates and the AAS derivatives allow the immune response of the organism. It is possible to obtain antisera with titers of 1/3000 to 1/100,000.

Naturally enough, the whole point is to choose the most expedient site on the AAS molecule for its binding to protein. Some people believe that the conjugation of a steroid with protein should be carried out through the molecular site which is furthest from the functional groups. This becomes relevant when obtaining antisera for natural androgens (testosterone, dihydrotestosterone, androsterone and others). Sometimes, when AAS and natural androgens are similar in structure and if they are of the same functional group, it is advisable to carry out the conjugation of AAS with protein only through these groups in order to reduce any cross reactivity with the natural steroid.

The evidence shows that when obtaining antisera for testosterone and 5α-dihydrotestosterone, as well as their conjugation with protein through positions 3, 6, 7 and 11, it is possible to obtain high specific antisera having only insignificant cross reactions with other hormones. The conjugations with protein through positions 3, 6, 7, and 11 are the most convenient and least labor-consuming for AAS. The keto group in position 3 of the steroid molecule is more available.

In our laboratory, a reliable and accessible method of obtaining conjugates of various AAS with BSA through position 3 of the steroid molecule ring A has been worked out. Figure 24 shows the formation of a peptide bond appearing as a result of the interaction of hapten carboxylmethyl-19-nortestosterone with free amino groups of BSA lysine radicals. By means of this method, the conjugates of seven AAS with BSA were obtained and their physical-chemical properties were studied. As a rule, the number of haptene molecules bound to an albumin molecule was within the limits of 20 to 30, which resulted in the effective use of immunogens during animal immunization. The evidence shows that if the position through which hapten is bound to protein is chosen correctly, it basically determines, with a high degree of specificity, the antisera for AAS.

The success of the immunization of animals depends on a number of factors. Among those that are worthy of note are molar relation of steroid-protein of the antigen used, conjugate doses, choice of adjuvant, and place and time of antigen injection. Animal selection for immunization is considered to be one of the most important moments for obtaining antisera. In the first experiments on obtaining antisera, sheep were used for the immunization.[21] In our experiments rabbits were used for carrying out the immunization and the antisera isolation for various AAS. Considerable differences between the animals and lack of special information on the intensity of antibody formation make the investigator's choice of the intervals between repeated immunogen injections somewhat empirical. The process of obtaining antisera should be considered to be the most time consuming and poorly controlled among all the steps in creating the method of AAS RIA. Although we have gained a great deal of experience in obtaining antisera for AAS, the truth is that the immune reactions of animals are strictly individual and the results of the immunization cannot always be precisely prognosticated. For example, Table 22 shows the order of steps carried out in the immunization of rabbits during the production of antisera for methandrostenolone which we use many times in our practice.

The evidence shows that when the antibody titer reaches its highest value, it starts gradually lowering. Considerable variations among animals are possible, and frequently in the application of maintained immunogen injections it is possible to retain a rather high titer. Figure 26 represents the scheme of rabbit immunization with BSA-methylandrostanediol conjugate. It can be seen that in 12 weeks an intensive formation of antibodies begins. It reaches the maximum value by the 17th week. Within this period the antibody titer makes up 1:6750. Then, 30, 33, and 36 weeks after the first immunization, reimmunization was done. However, as Figure 26 shows, the antibody titer obtained as a result of the reimmunization was lower (1:5500).

The antisera for androstane, androstene, and estrene AAS series for RIA were obtained, investigated, and used in our laboratory. Table 23 gives antisera titers of separate AAS for specimens of various series. One can see that the antisera obtained for various AAS had a titer within the limits of 5000 to 30,000, which allowed their use in RIA.

The presence of radioactively labeled AAS permitted the development of RIA

TABLE 22
Immunization Scheme (Obtaining the Antiserum Which Is Specific for Methandrostenolone)

1. Dissolve 1 mg of methandrostenolone conjugate with BSA in 0.5 ml of 0.4 M NaCl and add 0.5 ml of Freund adjuvant.
2. Inject the conjugates (1 ml) in small portions at the inner skin at four different points on the back of rabbit.
3. The injections are repeated once a week during 3 weeks.
4. Later on, the injections are repeated twice during 2 weeks.
5. A week after the last injection 2 ml of blood is taken for an examination, and then the immunization is maintained.

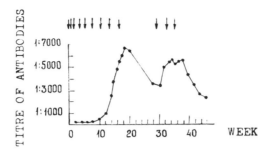

FIGURE 26. Scheme of rabbit immunization with BSA-methylandrostanediol conjugate. The arrows show the days of antigen injection.

for several steroid hormones including methandrostenolone, oxandrolone, methylandrostanediol, 19-nortestosterone, norethandrolone, testosterone, and estradiol.[22-29] It should be noted that AAS RIA is characterized by a high sensitivity and precision, sufficient specificity and practicality. For example, the RIA for methandrostenolone, one of the most widely used AAS,[30] was carried out by means of a direct method (without any extraction). The analysis used 0.3 ml of urine, and 0.1 ml of labeled hormone (7 to 9 pg) was introduced into each sample. Then the samples were mixed and 0.1 ml of antiserum was added. The samples were thoroughly remixed and incubated first at 37°C (for 30 min) and then at 4°C (for 15 min). Next, 0.5 ml of a cooled suspension of activated charcoal with dextran was added and the samples were incubated again at 4°C (for 10 min). Then, for 10 min the centrifugation of 3000 g of activated charcoal precipitate was carried out and 0.5 ml of the liquid was used for measuring the radioactivity. The results of the experiments show that by determining methandrostenolone in urine (without extraction) the linear dependence between the amount of the hormone contained in the urine sample and the initial hormone

TABLE 23
Comparison of Antisera Titers for
Various AAS

Series	Steroid	Titer
Androstane	Methylandrostanediol	1:6,750
	Oxandrolone	1:17,500
Androstene	Androstenediol	1:16,000
	Methandrostenolone	1:10,000
	Testosterone	1:30,000
Estrene	19-Nortestosterone	1:30,000
	Norethandrolone	1:5,000

concentration remained at a range in concentration of 15 to 150 pg of the hormone in the sample. The correlation coefficient was 0.99. The extraction of urine with ethyl ether showed the linear dependence between the amount of hormone contained in the sample and the hormone which was determined. Under these conditions, the sensitivity of the method made up 5.0 ± 0.7 pg. The reproduction of methandrostenolone RIA was investigated by multiple determinations of the content of the hormone, and variation within experiment was 4.9% and between experiments was 6.4%.

Although there has been quite a bit of success in using AAS RIA, it is necessary to note that this method has often been criticized for its insufficient specificity. As the evidence over these last few years has shown, there exist several real possibilities for increasing the specificity of RIA. One of them is associated with the use of column chromatography for isolating AAS from biological liquids with a subsequent application of RIA.[30] Another way, which is undoubtedly more perspective, attempts to obtain and use monoclonal antibodies in RIA.[31] Due to the great variety of AAS, which considerably differ in presence and location of diverse functional groups, the application of individual (monoclonal) antisera will lead to a considerable increase in their number and will complicate the analysis. A further perfection of AAS RIA is needed and there are three potential avenues:

1. Studying the possibility of using AAS labeled by various isotopes,
2. Obtaining and using polyclonal antisera for AAS groups, and
3. Selecting such parameters which are optimum for separate reagents of RIA and the automation of calculating the data for analysis.

To compare labeled ligands with inner and outer marks, an investigation on the possibility of using ^{3}H-19-nortestosterone and ^{125}I-19-nortestosterone in RIA was carried out.[32] The work was accomplished in the section of chemical pathology (Head — Prof. R. Brooks) at St. Thomas Hospital, London, England. They investigated some basic characteristics which the labeled ligands had to satisfy in RIA. The structures of labeled ^{3}H and ^{125}I-19-nortestosterone and the oxime conjugates of this hormone with BSA are given in Figure 27.

One can see that there are considerable differences in the location of the labeled isotope in the 19-nortestosterone molecule. By using ^{3}H the isotope is found in positions 6 and 7 of ring B inside the steroid molecule. In the case of ^{125}I, the isotope is bound to the steroid through 17-hemisuccinate and is situated outside the molecule. These differences in the location of the radioactive isotope make it possible to explain why there was not sufficient interaction between the antisera obtained for the conjugates of 3-(O-carboxymethyl)oxime of 19-nortestosterone-BSA and ^{125}I-19-nortestosterone (which was synthesized on the basis of 17-hemisuccinate of 19-nortestosterone) (Table 24).

The reason involves the absence of the structural conformity of the ligand with

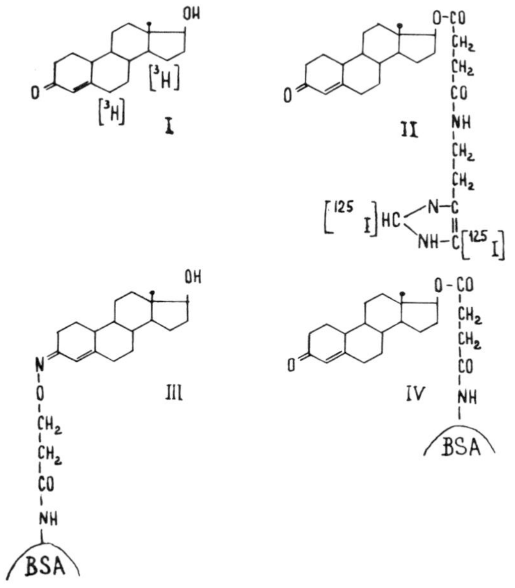

FIGURE 27. Structure of ³H-19-nortestosterone (I), ¹²⁵I-19-nortestosterone (II) and the conjugates 3-(O-carboxymethyl)-oxime 19-nortestosterone-protein (III) and 17-hemisuccinate 19-nortestosterone-protein (IV).

an outer radioactive mark to a steroid derivative for which the antiserum was obtained. It is known that antibodies are produced not only against haptene, but they also can recognize "the bridge" with the help of which the steroid is bound to protein. The absence of antibodies binding to ¹²⁵I-19-nortestosterone is obviously stipulated by the presence of "the bridge" which changes the stereochemical properties of a steroid molecule so that the antibodies, with a specificity to the steroid with the nonmodified ring D, cannot interact with such a hormone. Thus, the introduction of heterologous ¹²⁵I-steroid binding into the reaction can essentially affect the determination of AAS by means of RIA. One of the fundamental defects in the use of the outer ligand mark is manifested in this phenomenon. Such a problem cannot appear if a ligand with an inner mark ³H-AAS is used. In the experiments with (³H)-19-nortestosterone, the antiserum had a titer of 30,000, which made such labeled ligands more universal in AAS RIA. Comparison in the values of cross reactivity obtained for ³H and ¹²⁵I-19-nortestosterone did not reveal any essential differences. It has been established that the application of both tritium-labeled and iodinated steroids had no effect on the directivity of cross reactivities studied with six steroids. The sensitivity and the specificity of RIA in comparison with ³H and ¹²⁵I steroids proved to be similar according to their values (Table 24).

TABLE 24
Sensitivity of RIA for 19-Nortestosterone by
Using ^{125}I and ^{3}H Steroids

NN	Haptene	RIA sensibility (pg/ml)	
		^{125}I steroid	^{3}H steroid
1.	19-Nortestosterone-17-hemisuccinate-BSA	6.2	12.5
2.	19-Nortestosterone-3-(O-carboxymethyl)oxime-BSA	0	6.2

The comparison of AAS having an inner or outer radioactive marker and labeled by various isotopes led to the possibility of their application in AAS RIA.

Further investigations were directed at obtaining polyclonal antisera for AAS. As a rule, the investigator seeks to obtain a strictly specific antiserum, and in recent years monoclonal antibodies have been widely used for this reason. By using RIA for determining AAS it is quite reasonable to aim at not strict individual specificity, but rather at a group of antisera specificity in order to have cross reactions with a number of AAS having slight differences in their molecular structure.

What kinds of methods are available for obtaining antisera for AAS with a wide group specificity? At least two such approaches can be named. The first is associated with animal immunization by means of a specially compounded mixture of AAS conjugates with a homogenous protein such as with BSA. With this method it is possible to obtain a polyclonal antiserum of group specificity. The second method involves mixing several (2 to 3) individual antisera into the reaction mixture and analyzing by means of RIA. The possibility of using several antisera in one RIA reaction was shown in the example of 19-nortestosterone analysis, and apparently there are no principal obstacles for using such an approach for the analysis of AAS.[33]

In our laboratory we attempted to obtain a polyclonal antiserum for two or three AAS and compare the basic characteristics of such an antiserum with the mixture of individual antisera obtained for these AAS.[25,34]

During the selection of steroids for obtaining polyclonal antisera the principle of structural community was used. At the first stage of the work, 3-(O-carboxymethyl)oxime of methandrostenolone and 3-hemisuccinate of oxandrolone were synthesized. Then the conjugation of these substances with BSA using the carbodiimide method was carried out. The AAS conjugates obtained with protein had the same density as haptene (27 to 29 steroid molecules per albumin molecule). Following the scheme described above, the immunization of rabbits was carried out for 25 weeks. For the immunization different mixtures of conjugates were used:

1. Methylandrostanediol-BSA and methandrostenolone-BSA;
2. Methylandrostanediol-BSA, methandrostenolone-BSA and oxandrolone-BSA (1 mg each).

As a result of the immunization, two polyclonal antisera were obtained 25 weeks later. The first one had a titer of 1:6500 for methandrostenolone and 1:7500 for methylandrostanediol. The second one had a titer of 1:6450 for methandrostenolone, 1:6900 for methylandrostanediol, and 1:7200 for oxandrolone. In the course of immunization with the mixture of two conjugates and the mixture of three conjugates, the titer of antibodies was practically the same for each steroid. The polyclonal antisera obtained were used in RIA for determining sensitivity, specificity, and precision. The data on the determination of AAS RIA sensibility using the mixtures of individual and polyclonal antisera are given in Table 25. One can see that the polyclonal antisera determined the same AAS quantities as the mixture of individual antisera.

The comparison of precision of determination in RIA using polyclonal antisera and the mixture of individual antisera showed that they were not different.

The findings on antisera specificity are shown in Table 26. The table shows that all the antisera investigated have no cross reactions with natural steroids except androgens. The basic binding reactions are observed with AAS having a methyl group in the 17α position in their structure. The cross reactions for polyclonal antisera and the mixture of individual antisera appear to be similar. Higher cross reactions with a polyclonal antiserum were revealed only for separate steroids (methylandrostanediol, stanozolol, oxymetholone). The data obtained for determining the characteristics of polyclonal antisera show that they have a wide application in RIA based on the analysis of the content of AAS in human biological liquids.

In recent years, one of the principal trends in AAS RIA development has been the perfection of the method for the purpose of reducing the time and standardizing the analysis. It should be noted that in the first RIA for methandrostenolone it took 2 days to carry out the analysis. Working out the theoretical principles of

TABLE 25
RIA Sensitivity Using the Mixture of Individual and
Polyclonal Antisera (pg/Sample)

	Antisera			
Steroid	Polyclonal (I + II)	Mixture (I and II)	Polyclonal (I + II + III)	Mixture (I, II and III)
Methandrostenolone (I)	17 ± 0.8	17 ± 0.3	25 ± 0.9	25 ± 0.9
Methylandrostanediol (II)	33 ± 0.7	33 ± 0.8	50 ± 1.2	55 ± 1.3
Oxandrolone	—	—	100 ± 1.5	100 ± 1.6
Mixture I + II + III	25 ± 0.9	30 ± 1.1	50 ± 1.8	55 ± 1.3

TABLE 26
Cross Reactivity Using the Mixture of Individual
Antisera and Polyclonal Antisera (%)

NN	Steroid	Polyclonal antiserum for the mixture (I + II + III)	The mixture of individual antisera for I, II, III
1	2	3	4
1.	Mixture I + II + III	100	100
2.	Methandrostenolone (1)	158	163
3.	Methylandrostanediol (II)	68	71
4.	Oxandrolone (III)	48	39
5.	Methyltestosterone	161	170
6.	Mestanolone	107	109
7.	Stanozolol	25.3	24.1
8.	Oxymesterone	23.2	21
9.	Fluoxymesterone	10.3	9.8
10.	Mesterolone	1.3	1.2
11.	Metenolone	6.4	5.3
12.	19-Nortestosterone	2.3	2.2
13.	Oxymetholone	20.1	20.3
14.	Clostebol	0	0
15.	Norethandrolone	1.6	1.7
16.	Thiomesterone	9.3	7.6
17.	Lynesteronol	0	0
18.	Testosterone	24	23
19.	Dihydrotestosterone	15.9	15.1
20.	Ethyltestosterone	76	63
21.	Dihydroepiandrosterone	0	0
22.	Androstenediol	0.6	0.5
23.	Estriol	0	0
24.	Estradiol	0	0
25.	Progesterone	0	0
26.	Corticosterone	0	0
27.	Norethandrel	6.8	6.0
28.	Norethyldrone	16.4	18.1
29.	17β-Ethylestradiol	0	0

RIA, as well as the gradual increase in practical experience by different laboratories, led to a considerable reduction in the time of the analysis, chiefly due to a reduction in the time of sample incubation. A long period of sample incubation raises the possibility of steroid-antibody complex dissociation, which leads to a decrease in binding. There are also a number of technical difficulties in the laboratory itself which prevent wide use of RIA in clinical endocrinology. On the other hand, it turns out that the use of very short intervals of incubation time considerably increases the cross reactions of steroids.[35] The velocity of steroid-antibody complex dissociation plays a principal role in the determination of antisera specificity. The maximum specificity of antiserum may be achieved only by incubating under the conditions of equilibrium. It appears from this that to determine the minimum time of incubation in AAS RIA, the determination of the velocities of steroid-antibody complex association and dissociation is required. At present the possibility of a considerable decrease in incubation time using AAS RIA has been demonstrated by several laboratories.[33,36] Lately the problem of standardization of RIA conditions has become one of the most important issues. The problem is encountered when attempting to compare results obtained from commercial kits for RIA in different countries.

For this reason we carried out an investigation on the influence of various conditions of incubation in RIA for 19-nortestosterone. Principal attention was paid to reducing the sample incubation time, that is reducing the time of steroid-antibody complex interaction. As a result of the investigation the procedure for carrying out the reaction was to incubate 0.5 ml of steroid-antibody mixture for 30 min at 37°C and for 15 min at 0°C. Then we added equal volumes of dextran-charcoal suspension for separating free and bound antibodies with radioactive ^3H-19-nortestosterone and the samples were reincubated for 10 min at 0°C (RIA-1). By comparing this variant of determining 19-nortestosterone with another rapid procedure (RIA-2) used in one of the scientific centers (Department of Reproductive Endocrinology headed by Prof. E. Diszfalusy) at Karolina Institute, Stockholm, Sweden, it was shown that for obtaining 50% (^3H)-19-nortestosterone binding, it was necessary to use half of the antisera dilution in the RIA-2 system in comparison with RIA-1 (1:24,000 and 1:48,000, respectively).

The results of drawing calibration plots using the system of logit-log coordinates for 19-nortestosterone in various RIA systems are given at Table 27.

As the data in Table 27 show, the sensitivity, specificity, and some of the other characteristics of RIA for 19-nortestosterone essentially did not differ. There also were no considerable differences in the values of cross reactions of the antisera investigated with the eight various AAS. The findings on the precision and the reproduction of RIA for 19-nortestosterone showed that the coefficient of variation between the experiments made up 11.5%, within the experiment 7%, and the efficiency of 19-nortestosterone discovery 107.7%.

Thus, by comparing two variants of AAS RIA in the example of 19-nortestosterone, it was established that the value of antiserum dilution necessary for 50% of the radioactive steroid binding depends on the conditions of the analysis. It is of great significance when there are many analyses and considerable consumption of antisera. The results show that the practical application of this RIA variant for analyzing the content of 19-nortestosterone in biological liquids has potential. It is also apparent that by using RIA for determining other hormones, the estimation of its efficiency is needed so far as the optimal conditions of the reaction may be different.

Calculation of the analysis data, which until recently has been done by hand, plays an essential role in using AAS RIA today. From the results of data

TABLE 27
Calibrating Plot Characteristics Under Various
Conditions of 19-Nortestosterone RIA

19-Nortestosterone RIA	Sensitivity (pg/sample)	Incline value (B)	B_0/T (%)
RIA-1	6.25 ± 0.0	−2.35 ± 0.14	33.35 ± 3.25
RIA-2	6.25 ± 0.0	−2.31 ± 0.19	37.70 ± 14.81

calculations, a calibration plot was produced and led to a wider application of small desktop calculators. A number of methods allowed the transformation of the calibration plots into a linear form. The theoretical grounds and practical use of logit-log was offered by Rodbord.[37-39] At present a number of approximative functions for AAS RIA data calculation are used. They may be divided into two main classes: linear and nonlinear approximations. Linear logit-log analysis remains one of the most widely used methods of experimental data approximation due to the simplicity of its processing.

The logit value is calculated according to the following formula:

$$\log \text{it} \quad b = \lg_e\left(\frac{b}{100 - b}\right) \tag{10}$$

where b is the constant of the labeled steroid in bound form and is expressed as a percentage of its content in zero standard. The plot of the dependence of this value versus the logarithm of concentration gives a direct line. The use of this value in making the program of a linear regression of the smallest squares for small desktop calculators completely automates the data calculations. For this reason and by drawing up the mathematical models we used the minicomputer "Electronics D 3-28" in our work. The use of logit-log analysis has a number of limitations due to the presence of nonlinearity, and while using polyclonal antisera one will often come across this phenomenon. The linearization of the problem in carrying out an experiment, under real conditions, leads to a distortion of the sensitivity of the method. The use of a nonlinear dependence in the logit-log analysis cannot be recognized as one of the best ways of the approximation either since not veritable but transformed data obtained in the experiment are analyzed, which gives some additional errors during the calculations.

The logical approximation or the "four-parameter function" is used most seldom because of the complexity of the calculations. The given methodological approach for the processing of RIA data for methandrostenolone and 19-nortestosterone was used in our laboratory.[40]

The experimental data approximation using the four-parameter function becomes:

$$B = \frac{B_0 - B_N}{1 + \left(\dfrac{DD}{ED_{50}} \right)^b} + BN \qquad (11)$$

where B is response in dpm/min, B_0 is the coefficient characterizing the initial binding, B_N is the coefficient characterizing the nonspecific binding, D is the dose determined in pg/mg, ED_{50} is the midpoint of the dose-response curve, and b is the coefficient characterizing the steepness of the curve. The calculation of the coefficients B_0 and B_N[37,39] and knowledge of the regularity of their changes are also needed. Until now there has been no information about how to determine, in a rapid and most favorable way, the values of the basic reagents of AAS RIA, a radioactive steroid, antiserum for steroid, and activated charcoal (mostly used for separating free and bound fractions) for obtaining trustworthy and repeatable results. In practice it is usually carried out by means of numerous experiments and depends to a large extent on the intuition of the investigator. We have worked out a methodological approach that will estimate the values of the basic parameters of steroid RIA on the basis of carrying out the two-factor experiment by an express method when high precision and reliable analysis of the data are ensured. We could say that in fact we are examining the problem on the basis of the association between P, P^x and Q components in the reaction of RIA:

$$P + Q \rightleftharpoons PQ$$
$$P^x + Q \rightleftharpoons P^x Q \qquad (12)$$

where P^x is a radioactive steroid, P is a nonradioactive steroid, and Q is an antibody.

The change in the association between the concentration of P^x, P and Q influences the values of both B_0 and B_N. Figure 28 represents the function corresponding to Equation 11 where the value B characterizes the count of radioactivity for the concentration of steroid P and the value of B_0 is the count of radioactivity obtained when P = 0. A precise definition of B_0 and B_N as well as the coefficient ED_{50} and the value characterizing the deviation of the standard curve which is dependent on them gives an approximative function of the type in Equation 11 with a small quadratic deviation from experimental data. Study of the changes in mean values and the dispersions of B_0 and B_N from the values of principal RIA parameters makes it possible to carry out an experiment that determines their optimum values. This leads to the highest precision and reliability of the data.

As a criterion for the optimum choice of principal parameters of AAS RIA, a minimum dispersion of the standard dose-response curve was used. The dispersion value of the standard curve may be represented as the sum of contributions of the following values:

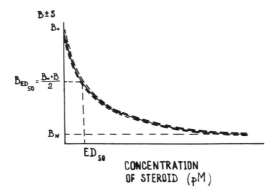

FIGURE 28. Typical standard curve: methandrostenolone assay. B_0, a count of radioactivity for a zero dose; B_N, a count of radioactivity of a nonspecific binding; ED_{50}, a dose of 50% binding; S, standard deviation of value B.

- Dispersion characterizing the purity of the reagents used and the heterogeneity of their properties which is a matter of a preliminary estimate;
- Dispersion characterizing a variance by nonspecific binding in the RIA reaction;
- Dispersion characterizing a variance in the reaction of specific binding — steroid-antibody.

Hence, one can distinguish two basic factors affecting the value of dispersion of the standard dose-response curve in the AAS RIA reaction, a specific and a nonspecific steroid binding.

To simplify the conditions of carrying out the two-factor experiment and to rapidly find optimum values of principal AAS RIA parameters, we made a supposition about the independence of these two factors. Later on such a supposition found experimental and quantitative confirmation by calculation of the value of the correlation coefficient between the parameters of the standard curve (which characterize a specific and nonspecific binding effect). The problem of nonspecific binding (B_N) is considered to be one of the most important problems. This is because of the presence of an error in dividing free and bound fractions which exerts an essential influence on the reliability of the data during the RIA reaction. The factors influencing the value of nonspecific binding are examined in detail in a number of works.[1,4,41] Among them we could distinguish the presence of substances in samples which prevent the interaction of the antiserum with steroid, dissociation of labeled steroid, antiserum inactivation, and variance of free sample.[42-44] The factor of nonspecificity appears to be more significant in the determination of the optimum values of the principal parameters of RIA. An optimum choice of radioactive steroid values and the activated charcoal concentrations achieve a high specificity in the process of minimizing nonspecific binding in the RIA reaction.

In the first stage of carrying out the two-times experiment for finding the optimum concentrations of activated charcoal and radioactive ligand, we used the methodologies worked out in our laboratory.[40] We determined the dependence of the error in dividing free and bound fractions ($F = B_N/T\%$) and the variation ($C_v = S_{BN}/B_N\%$) in the reaction of nonspecific steroid binding on the concentrations of activated charcoal and radioactive steroid.[45] In this case, we found the concentration of activated charcoal corresponding to the minimum values of C_v and F. For a selected optimum charcoal concentration, we plotted the dependence of F and C_v on T and determined the range of optimum values of T according to the minimum C and the minimum admissible value of F. The full precipitation of labeled ligand by the activated charcoal is an ideal result of nonspecific binding in AAS RIA. In this case, the variation of B_N must be minimized and appears to be a criterion for the stability of the given reaction. The analysis of the error value for the division of free and bound fractions showed that if the concentration of the activated charcoal rose, the value of F was reduced and reached low values.

The optimum values of the charcoal concentration were chosen according to the values of the total radioactivity (T). It has been established that a charcoal concentration of 0.5% is critical for methandrostenolone in the range of mean and low values of T (T << 7200 dpm/min) while for 19-nortestosterone it is in the range of mean values (T = 7000 dpm/min). By using the critical charcoal concentration, a great variation in the estimation of standard curve dispersion is observed which leads to reliable differences between analyses with the same values of RIA basic parameters. Analysis of the findings leads to the hypothesis that by carying out RIA for methandrostenolone and 19-nortestosterone, the use of charcoal in a concentration of 1.0% leads to relatively small errors in the division of free and bound fractions. In the end, certain values of total radioactivity give the possibility of obtaining a small variation in the value of B_N.

For the chosen value of the charcoal concentration, C_v and F dependence on the value of the total radioactivity (T) was plotted. Figure 29 represents the ranges of the optimum values of T as a hatched region for determining methandrostenolone and 19-nortestosterone. In the case of T, for great values of these steroids, a reliable difference between the experiments may appear. Thus, it is always necessary to qualitatively control the given experiment.

The next step in determining the basic parameters of AAS RIA in the rapid method is to obtain the optimum conditions for a specific binding steroid-antibody. Using well-known methods[46] we drew up the plots to find the antiserum dilution corresponding to its maximum capability (F) for a certain interval of unlabeled steroid concentration. Figure 30 represents an example of the curves of antisera capability in RIA for methandrostenolone according to the value of initial binding (B_0/T) and the concentration of unlabeled methandro-

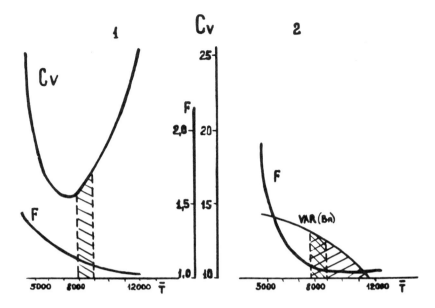

FIGURE 29.   Determination of optimum value of steroid total radioactivity: 1 — methandrostenolone; 2 — 19-nortestosterone.

stenolone. The function F^i of an antiserum with i-dilution is calculated as the difference in the ratio of average values of the initial binding for some concentrations of unlabeled steroid ($\overline{B}_0^i$) to the value of their error:

$$F^i = \frac{\overline{B}_0^i - \overline{B}_p^i}{\sqrt{(\Delta_0^i) + (\Delta_p^i)^2}} \tag{13}$$

As Figure 30 shows, the value of antisera capability essentially depends on the determined concentration of steroid which stipulates the choice of the initial binding value. For RIA of methandrostenolone and 19-nortestosterone in the range of 25 to 200 pg in a sample, the optimum values of antisera initial binding for methandrostenolone make up 54 to 62% and for 19-nortestosterone 45 to 55%. By using the antisera for 19-nortestosterone, a two-bent character of the curve was revealed. Thus, in the example of two AAS, it was shown that the choice of optimum values of the RIA basic parameters is a necessary condition for obtaining precise and reliable data.

Improving the quality of AAS RIA is thus closely connected with obtaining antiserum and labeled ligand, sample preparation for the analysis, reagent dispersion, division of free and bound radioactivity, quality control, and standardization of procedures. An analysis of RIA technological operations showed

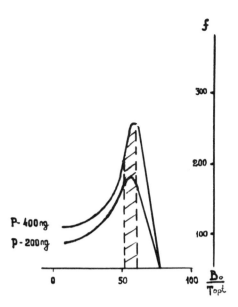

FIGURE 30. Determination of optimum value of
methandrostenolone antisera initial binding.

that there are 44 indices which, to a certain extent, influence the final result.[47]
Knowing that, attention should be paid to the technique of carrying out the
analysis, the precision of pipetting, the reproducibility of the result, etc. To
control the RIA quality inside the laboratory, it is important to achieve constant
indices of maximum (B_0) parameters and minimum (nonspecific) binding as
well as an admissible variation of the control specimen.

The problem of statistical analysis and automated processing of AAS RIA data
is linked to the major problems that investigators meet while using this method
in clinical biochemistry. A great deal of attention should be paid to a dispersed
estimation of RIA standard curves and the effect of casual mistakes by technical
staff, for instance during pipetting.[44,46,47] By analysis of such mistakes one can
sort out the values of basic parameters of dose-response curves so that the value
of errors and the consequence of this on the dispersion curve could be considerably reduced. The use of dispersed models also can control RIA qualitatively. By
AAS RIA optimum planning, two factors affecting the course of the reaction
were examined: nonspecific binding (B_N) and initial binding (B_0/T).[40]

The experiments carried out showed that the nature of the dispersed curve for
19-nortestosterone and methandrostenolone antisera represents a curve of the
second order:

$$S^2 = B_0^2 \cdot C_0 + C_1 \cdot B_0 \cdot B + C_2 B \tag{14}$$

where S^2 is a square of standard curve dispersion, B_0 is an initial binding, and C_0, C_1, C_2 are coefficients of the dispersed curve.

The change in values of nonspecific and initial binding influence the values of minimum and maximum dispersion of the standard curve. By drawing statistically averaged models of AAS RIA standard curves, we used the method of planning extreme experiments to estimate the values investigated with maximum truth. Figure 31 gives averaged dispersion curves for 19-nortestosterone and methandrostenolone antisera, the coefficients of dispersed curves, and their errors. A curve of the second order was used for 19-nortestosterone as the description of the dispersed model. The data showed that this aspect of the dispersed curve had a more complicated character. To draw the dispersed models we determined the regions of working doses obtained by the analysis of the distribution of AAS concentrations in biosamples.

For approximating RIA standard curves using polyclonal antisera for AAS, the choice of more complicated functions is needed. In this case, the following logical function may be used:[48]

$$B = \frac{b_0}{1 + b_1 \cdot \exp(a_0 + a_1 t + \ldots a_n t)} \tag{15}$$

where b_0, b_1, a_0, and a_1 are parameters and t is the time.

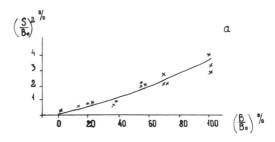

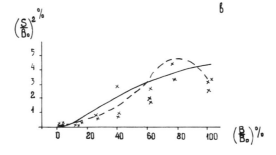

FIGURE 31.   Dispersed estimates of standard curves of methandrostenolone (a) and 19-nortestosterone (b) RIA.

The use of standard curves for the functions of the kind in Equation 15 for approximating experimental data enables a more complete optimization of AAS RIA when not only specific antisera, but also polyclonal antisera with a group specificity, are used.

At present, for mathematical analysis of RIA data, different approaches using a small desktop calculators are used, which completely automates the calculations.[49,52] In our laboratory to analyze the AAS RIA data we used a microcomputer, "Electronics D 3-28", and a program including about 6000 bits was written.[53] A simplified block scheme of this program is given in Figure 32.

For building a standard curve and analyzing the samples, the following AAS RIA parameters are introduced into the computer:

1. Number of points of standard curve (m);
2. Number of standard and control sample patterns (n ≥ m);
3. Value of steroid concentration in standard curve samples;
4. Multiples of standard and control samples;
5. Account of standard and control patterns;
6. Coefficients of dispersed model;
7. Number of samples analyzed;
8. Number of recount in pg/ml;
9. Critical dose of response;
10. Data on samples analyzed: multiple and the count of samples patterns.

By building the standard curve in analytic form, the Newton-Gauss modified suspended method of least squares for the case of nonlinear dependence on the

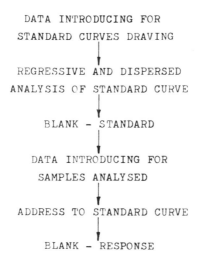

DATA INTRODUCING FOR
STANDARD CURVES DRAVING

↓

REGRESSIVE AND DISPERSED
ANALYSIS OF STANDARD CURVE

↓

BLANK – STANDARD

↓

DATA INTRODUCING FOR
SAMPLES ANALYSED

↓

ADDRESS TO STANDARD CURVE

↓

BLANK – RESPONSE

FIGURE 32. Simplified block scheme for AAS RIA automatic processing.

parameters was used. In the process of theoretical curve approximation to the experimental data, the gravimetric functions, inversely proportional to the dispersion squares of the values observed, were used. Their use resulted in precise estimates of parameters and their errors. First information on standard samples is introduced into the Ec and the data on its processing (theoretical curve, its coefficient of regressive curve, and the concentration of control samples) are typed onto a blank standard. Then information for unknown samples is introduced. After the processing of this information, the data are given on the blank response where there is an average concentration of the samples, its variance in the range of two standard derivatives, and the result of a parallelism test.

The analysis of dispersed estimates of the coefficients of the standard curve dispersion regressions and those of the correlative matrix allows for qualitative control of AAS RIA.

The creation of the system of mathematical analysis, as well as the program of automated processing of AAS RIA, not only provides our laboratory with the ability to carry out serial analyses, but also increases the precision and reliability of the data obtained.

REFERENCES

1. **Chard, T.,** *An Introduction to Radioimmunoassay and Related Techniques,* North-Holland, Amsterdam, 1978.
2. **Tkatscheva, G. A., Balaboyakin, M. I., and Laritscheva, I. P.,** Radioimmunochemical methods of investigation, *Medicine,* Moscow, 1983.
3. **Joffe, B. M. and Behrnan, H. R., Eds.,** *Methods of Hormone Radioimmunoassay,* Academic Press, New York, 1979.
4. **Vining, R. F.,** Steroid radioimmunoassay, *Clin. Biochem. Rev.,* 2, 39, 1981.
5. **Parker, C. W.,** Radioimmunoassay, *Annu. Rev. Pharm. Toxicol.,* 21, 113, 1982.
6. **Hampl, R. and Starek, L.,** Labeled steroid compounds, *Radioisotopy,* 19, 337, 1978.
7. **Johnson, D. W., Phillipou, G., and Seamark, R. F.,** Deuterium labeled steroid hormones: synthesis and applications in quantitative endocrinology, *J. Steroid Biochem.,* 14, 793, 1981.
8. **Hampl, R., Dvorak, P., Lukesova, S., Koza, K. I., Chrpova, M., and Starka, L.,** The use of iodinated steroid as radioligand for testosterone radioimmunoassay, *J. Steroid Biochem.,* 9, 771, 1978.
9. **Ignatjeva, N. A., Tatarkina, F. V., Kaklyshkina, L. N., Tupizin, I. E., and Mishin, V. I.,** Tritium labelled anabolic steroids used for radioimmunoassay. I. Synthesis of 19-nortestosterone-(6,7³H), 17α-ethyl-19-nortestosterone-(6,7³H) and 1-dehydro-17α-methyltestosterone-(6,7³H), in *Medical and Doping Control of Athletes,* Leningrad, 1981, 80.
10. **Rogozkin, V. A. and Tschaikovsky, V. S.,** Radioimmunoassay — a method of screening-analysis of anabolic steroids, in *Medical and Doping Control of Athletes,* Leningrad, 1981, 27.
11. **Schall, R. F. and Tenoso, H. S.,** Alternation to radioimmunoassay: labels and methods, *Clin. Chem.,* 27, 1157, 1981.
12. **Koen, F., Linder, H. R., and Gilad, S.,** Development of chemiluminescence monitored immunoassays for steroid hormones, *J. Steroid Biochem.,* 19, 413, 1983.

165

13. **Exley, D.,** Steroid immunoassay in clinical chemistry, *Pure Appl. Chem.,* 52, 33, 1979.
14. **Hampl, R., Stolla, P., Putz, Z., Protiva, J., Kimlova, L., and Starka, L.,** Advances in immunoassay of anabolic steroids, in *Radioimmunoassay and Related Procedures in Medicine,* Proc. Int. Symp., Vienna, June 21 to 25, 1982, 365.
15. **Erlander, B. F., Beiser, S. M., and Borek, F.,** The preparation of steroid-protein conjugates to elicit autohormonal antibodies, in *Methods in Immunology and Immunochemistry,* Williams, I. C. A. and Chase, E., Eds., Academic Press, New York, 1967, 144.
16. **Dean, P. D. C., Exley, D., and Johnson, M. W.,** Preparation of 17-oestradiol-6-(o-carboxymethyl-3)oxime-bovine serum albumin conjugate, *Steroids,* 18, 593, 1971.
17. **Linder, H. R., Perol, E., Fridlander, A., and Zeitlin, A.,** Specificity of antibodies to ovarian hormone in relation to the site of attachment of the steroid hapten to the peptide carrier, *Steroids,* 19, 357, 1972.
18. **Morozov, V. I. and Tschaikovsky, V. S.,** Radioimmunoassay as a screening analysis of anabolic steroid, in *Muscular Activity and Hormones,* Leningrad, 1982, 18.
19. **Midgley, A. R., Hiswender, G. D.,** Radioimmunoassay of steroids, *Acta Endocrinol.,* 64, 320, 1970.
20. **Abraham, G. E.,** Radioimmunoassay of steroids in biological materials, *Acta Endocrinol.,* 75, 7, 1974.
21. **Brooks, R., Firth, R., and Summer, N.,** Detection of anabolic steroids by radioimmunoassay, *Br. J. Sports Med.,* 9, 89, 1975.
22. **Rogozkin, V. A., Tschaikovsky, V. S., and Morosov, V. I.,** Method of radioimmunoassay for methandrostanolone in urine, *Chem. Pharmacol. J.,* N4, 98, 1979.
23. **Rogozkin, V. A., Morosov, V. I., and Tschaikovsky, V. S.,** Rapid radioimmunoassay for anabolic steroids in urine, *Schweiz. Zeitschr. Sportmed.,* 4, 169, 1979.
24. **Tschaikovsky, V. S., Morosov, V. I., and Rogozkin, V. A.,** Method of radioimmunoassay for the determination of steroids in biological fluids, in *Medicine and Sports,* Leningrad, 1979, 130.
25. **Tschaikovsky, V. S., Morosov, V. I., and Rogozkin, V. A.,** Radioimmunoassay of anabolic steroids: possibilities and perspective, in *Doping Control of Athletes,* Moscow, 1980, 95.
26. **Rogozkin, V. A. and Tschaikovsky, V. S.,** Radioimmunoassay — a method of screening analysis of anabolic steroids, in *Medical and Doping Control of Athletes,* Leningrad, 1981, 27.
27. **Tadzhiev, F. S., Morosov, V. I., and Rogozkin, V. A.,** Radioimmunoassay for methylandrostendiol in biological liquids, *Immunology (USSR),* 2, 89, 1982.
28. **Tschaikovsky, V. S. and Morosov, V. I.,** Radioimmunoassay for anabolic steroids, *Sci. Rev. Univ. Tartu,* 606, 121, 1982.
29. **Tschaikovsky, V. S., Zorina, A. D., Korneva, I. A., and Rogozkin, V. A.,** Testosterone content in human biological liquids by different methods of introducing into organism, *Probl. Endocrinol. (USSR),* N4, 39, 1983.
30. **Bosch, A.,** A radioimmunoassay of 19-nortestosterone using celite column chromatography, *J. Clin. Chem. Clin. Biochem.,* 22, 29, 1984.
31. **Fantl, V. E. and Wang, D. Y.,** Characterization of monoclonal antibodies raised against testosterone, *J. Steroid Biochem.,* 19, 1605, 1983.
32. **Morosov, V. I. and Tschaikovsky, V. S.,** Radioimmune screen-analysis of anabolic steroids, in *Muscular Activity and Hormones,* Leningrad, 1982, 18.
33. **Hampl, R. and Starka, L.,** Practical aspects of screening of anabolic steroids in doping control with particular accent to nortestosterone radioimmunoassay using mixed antiserum, *J. Steroid Biochem.,* 11, 933, 1979.
34. **Morosov, V. I. and Tadzhiev, F. S.,** Polyvalent antiserum for methandrostenolone and methylandrostendiol and the capabilities of its application for doping control, in *Medical and Doping Control of Athletes,* Leningrad, 1981, 56.
35. **Vining, R. F., Compton, P., and McGinley, R.,** Steroid radioimmunoassay: effect of shortened incubation time on specificity, *Clin. Chem.,* 27, 920, 1981.

36. **Brooks, R. V., Hooper, H., and Webb, W. A.,** Detection of anabolic steroid administration by radioimmunoassay, in *Doping Control of Athletes,* Moscow, 1980, 105.

37. **Rodbard, D., Ruder, H., and Vaitukaitis, I.,** Mathematical analysis of kinetics of radioligand assays, *J. Clin. Endocrinol. Metabol.,* 33, 343, 1971.

38. **Rodbard, D.,** Statistical quality control and routine data processing for radioimmunoassays and immunoradiometric assays, *Clin. Chem.,* 20, 1255, 1974.

39. **Rodbard, D.,** Statistical estimation of the minimal detectable concentration for radioligand assays, *Anal. Biochem.,* 90, 1, 1978.

40. **Korneva, J. A. and Ivanova, E. M.,** Estimation of the main optimal parameters of steroid radioimmunoassay, in *Medical and Doping Control of Athletes,* Leningrad, 1981, 41.

41. **Abraham, G.,** Radioimmunoassay of steroids in biological fluids, *J. Steroid Biochem.,* 6, 261, 1975.

42. **Abraham, G. E., Manlinnos, F. S., and Garza, R.,** RIA of steroids, in *Handbook of RIA,* Abraham, G. E., Ed., Marcel Dekker, New York, 1977, 591.

43. **Gekan, S. L.,** On the assessment of validity of steroid RIA, *J. Steroid Biochem.,* 11, 1629, 1979.

44. **Schinde, J., Jacker, R. R., Ntunde, B., and Smith, V. G.,** Steroid radioimmunoassays: the problems of blanks, *Can. J. Anim. Sci.,* 61, 363, 1981.

45. **Korneva, I. A. and Tschaikovsky, V. S.,** Effect of the conditions of dividing free and bound ligands on the accuracy of steroids radioimmunoassay, *Vopr. Med. Chem. (USSR),* 30, 122, 1984.

46. **Thorell, J. S. and Larson, S. M.,** *Radioimmunoassay and Related Techniques, Methodology and Clinical Application,* C. V. Mosby, St. Louis, 1978.

47. **Levada, M., Safarcik, K., and Topglcan, O.,** Some problems of radioimmunoassay control, *J. Radioanal. Chem.,* 46, 57, 1978.

48. **Venetsky, I. G.,** Statistic method in domography, *Statistics,* Moscow, 1977, 51.

49. **Metta, M., Bono, G., and Bolellio, G.,** Mathematical analysis of antiserum titer and affinity in rabbits injected with 11α-hydroxyprogesterone hemisuccinate-BSA, *J. Steroid Biochem.,* 7, 19, 1976.

50. **Cernosek, S. F. and Gutierrez-Cernosek, R. M.,** Use of a programmable desk-top calculator for the statistical quality control of radioimmunoassays, *Clin. Chem.,* 24, 1121, 1978.

51. **Raab, M.,** Comparison of a logistic and a mass-action curve for radioimmunoassay data, *Clin. Chem.,* 29, 1757, 1983.

52. **Wilkins, T. A.,** Comparison of a logistic and a mass-action curve for radioimmunoassay, *Clin. Chem.,* 30, 585, 1984.

53. **Korneva, I. A. and Tschaikovsky, V. S.,** Mathematic analysis in automatic processing of the results of anabolic steroids radioimmunoassay, in *Medical and Doping Control of Athletes,* Leningrad, 1981, 48.

Chapter 9

CHROMATOGRAPHIC METHODS OF
AAS DETERMINATION

At present about 100 various AAS and a considerable number of their metabolites are known. As a rule, after a single or systematic injection their content in organic liquids and tissues is extremely low in comparison with endogenic steroid hormones. It is necessary to bear in mind that there are also a great variety of endogenous steroid hormones and their metabolites. Suffice it to say that only in human urine have scientists successfully isolated and identified more than 100 various steroids by means of physical-chemical methods. These circumstances led to a considerable expansion of up-to-date physical-chemical methods which are used for AAS analysis. To isolate AAS from biological liquids, different methods of chromatographic analysis are available, such as partition, adsorption, ion-exchange and gel chromatography in different forms — column, paper, thin-layer on plates, and gas chromatography (GC), both separately and in combination with each other. In general, the application of these chromatographic methods is described in detail in a number of monographs.[1-4] In this chapter we will dwell only on those which have direct application to AAS analysis.

The theoretical foundations of partition chromatography used in columns, on paper, thin-layer on plates or GC are linked to the same principles as those used in adsorption chromatography. However, when these methods are used for steroid separation, there are essential differences.

Column chromatography may be divided into two general types, partition and adsorption chromatography. The advantage of column chromatography is the possibility of dividing large amounts of steroid mixtures without overloading the system, which is impossible when using thin-layer or paper chromatography. The change in the size of the column used is reflected by the efficiency of steroid separation. The division of steroids which are similar in structure depends on the efficiency of the selected chromatographic system. This may be determined by the size of sorbent particles and the ratio of length to width of the column. When the width of the column increases without an accompanying increase in length, efficiency is reduced. These questions are described in more detail in Reference 3.[3]

Partition column chromatography uses many systems of solvents, which are based primarily on the mixture of organic solvents with hydrous alcohols. The water stationary phase is bound to celite in the column. They are usually used in portions of 0.5 to 0.7 parts of stationary phase to one part of celite (by weight). Then celite washed by stationary phase is mixed with mobile phase and packed in the column. After packing, the top of the column is covered with the steroid mixture as a narrow stripe and then eluted by means of a mobile phase under pressure. The latter is made by a liquid in a reservoir which is situated at the top of the column. The steroids present in the mixture are distributed according to the size of different mobilities between mobile and stationary phases. The complete division of all the steroids present in biological liquids requires the use of several systems. After passing through the column, the mobile phase is collected and the concentration of steroids can be determined either by means of ultraviolet absorption or with the help of a colored reaction.

The investigation of various factors that influence the velocity and effectiveness of dividing the columns led to the development of high-phase liquid chromatography (HPLC). In recent years considerable progress in the field of HPLC theory and the creation of columns, detectors, and other equipment has been achieved. It has made this method as accessible in laboratory practice as GC.[5] The application of HPLC in AAS analysis has been especially beneficial because the limitation associated with a low volatility of these combinations, typical of GC, is not a problem for HPLC. This considerably simplifies and expedites the preparation and analysis of samples. Another advantage of this method, which is no less important, is the possibility of analyzing the conjugate forms of steroids using glucuronic or sulphuric acids.[6,7]

The principal questions of the application of HPLC for AAS determination have been examined in detail.[8] The possibility of increasing the sensitivity and selectivity of HPLC is associated with using a fluorescent and electrochemical detector which leads to the use of small packing and glass capillary columns.

Comparing the possibilities of HPLC with gas chromatography (GC), it should be noted that in liquid chromatography, in addition to the change in polarity of the stationary phase, it is also possible to change the polarity of the mobile phase. This fact considerably increases the possibilities of HPLC in comparison with other methods used for AAS analysis. In our laboratory, we have achieved a satisfactory division of testosterone, epitestosterone, and 19-nortestosterone in column with converted phase RP-18.[8] As Figure 33 shows, we succeeded in separating these substances and determined their concentration for a short period of time.

Today HPLC is more frequently used for determining androgens and AAS in human biological liquids, mainly with the use of columns with converted phases.[9] It should be noted that the successful use of columns with such stationary phases as nonpolar octadecylsilyl and more polar phases containing end nitrile groups has been accomplished. In these conditions, a clear separation of methandienone and its derivatives occurs. The possibility of their quantitative determination within the limits of 1 to 5 ng in a sample has been shown.[10]

Selica gels containing diphenylsilyl groups may be used as carriers as well. It was shown that the retention of steroids on the silica gel surface modified by diphenylchlorosilane from water-ethanol phases was determined by the ratio of hydrophilic to hydrophobic groups in a steroid molecule.[11] The possibility of a rapid and accurate separation of seven testosterone metabolites was accomplished by means of HLPC. The application of a three-component mixture (methanol-water-acetonitrite) for the elution resulted in good efficiency of all the

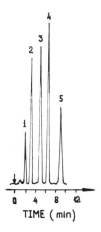

FIGURE 33. Chromatogram of steroid mixture on ODZ-HC-SIL-X-1 (0.26 × 25 cm) 30% acetonitrile solvent at 1 ml/min; the absorbance was read at 254 nm. Peaks: 1, cortisol; 2, corticosterone; 3, 19-nortestosterone; 4, testosterone; 5, epitestosterone.

metabolites.[12] The combination of HPLC methods with RIA is possible. Using this combination one can quantitatively determine the content of basic androgens and their metabolites in blood. In the first stage the separation of blood extract in the column with converted phase (C-18) in a methanol-water system is carried out. The quantitative determination of each steroid fraction is accomplished by using RIA.[13] Attempts to use the GC method for AAS analysis did not prove to be as numerous and successful. One of the main reasons which delays a more extensive application of GC is associated with technical complications which appear during the analysis. First of all, it is necessary to convert steroids to a volatile state so that the substances analyzed may leave the column in the form of narrow peaks and not have a residual or nonreversible adsorption. For this reason different methods of modifying the polar functional groups of the steroid are used, such as silylation, acetylation, and others. It should be noted that the number of AAS in human biological liquids is considerably lower in comparison with the content of natural androgens, which also creates some technical difficulties. For a long time packing columns were used for steroid analysis. However, the efficiency of such columns was too low for the analysis of multicomponent biological liquids. Recently a considerable increase in column efficiency and the diminution of the values of residual adsorption (especially by using flexible capillary columns made of melted quartz) have led to an essential improvement in the results of the analysis of steroids.[15-17]

The creation of an indivisible chromato-mass-spectrometric system (GC-MS) greatly extended the possibilities of the analysis of separating difficult mixtures of organic substances.[18] The joining of the mass spectrometer to GC gives a highly perceptible and specific detector that can identify the components of mixtures introduced into the chromatograph. The basis of the method consists of subjecting the substance under investigation to ionization in a mass spectrometer. It is then divided into ion bundles having the same ratio of mass to charge and their number is recorded. Most frequently the ionization of substances is made in a gaseous state. The most widespread method of AAS ionization is the use of electronic impact. Electronic impact is an interaction of substance molecules with the electron flow, which leads to the excitation of the molecular electronic envelope and the removal of one of the electrons. The other kind of ionization used is chemical ionization. It mainly consists of an initial ionization by electronic impact of a gas reactant which later interacts with the molecules of the substance analyzed. Other methods of ionization, such as photoionization and field ionization, have not yet been practiced in AAS analysis. The ions are distributed according to masses which are necessary for obtaining a mass spectrum. It is based on the ions differing in the mass ratio to the charge (m/e) in electronic and magnetic field. Mass spectra enables not only identification of the substance analyzed, but also its quantitative determination. According to ion separation, magnetic and quadripolar mass spectrometers have been used on a large scale. With the application of mass fragmentography using magnetic spectrometers it is possible to determine substances in picogram (10^{-12}) quantities one to two orders higher than by using detectors which are usually used in GC. Mass fragmentography has the largest use in the qualitative and quantitative analysis of various medicines (and their metabolites) which are in a complex mixture with natural metabolites in an organism.[19,20] The high sensitivity of the method can determine the substances and their metabolites which are introduced into the organism in therapeutic doses and the high specificity gives the possibility of analyzing complex mixtures. There are a number of reviews where the possibility of using this method for the analysis of steroid hormones is examined in more detail.[21-24] Just as in GC, the choice of column phases and the type of derivatives play an essential role. One of the most tedious, but necessary, tasks the investigator must resolve in AAS analysis is considered to be careful preparation of biosamples for their introduction into the GC-MS system.

To isolate steroids from various biological liquids, ion-exchange chromatography with diverse sorbents is used. At first there were different types of resins used for concentrating the biosamples and purifying the steroids from chromogens which prevent colorimetric determination.[25,26] It turned out that the steroid losses associated with nonspecific adsorption made it difficult to use these resins in quantitative analysis. The appearance of DEAE-Sephadex with a low nonspecific sorbing with respect to steroids permitted them to be used for isolating steroids.[27] Columns with DEAE-Sephadex in a chloride form began to be used with a subsequent elution of steroids and sodium chloride. An advantage of ion-exchange chromatography is that with the appearance of lyophilized derivatives of di- and tetraethylaminohydroxypropyl (DEAP-LH-20; TEAP-LH-20), there appeared the possibility of separating the steroids into groups containing free hormones, monoglucuronides, monosulphates, and disulphates.[28-31]

When preparing biosamples containing AAS for analysis on a GC-MS system, it is necessary to consider the fact that most steroids are present in the conjugate form with glucuronic or sulphuric acid. To determine these conjugate forms a preliminary enzymic or acidic hydrolysis is needed. Thus, preparation of the samples takes much more time than analysis on the mass spectrometer. Hence, there appears the necessity for improving the technique of sample preparation for analysis in order to reduce the time for performing this operation. In our laboratory we studied in detail a few stages in the preparation of samples containing AAS for analysis using GC-MS. First we investigated the possibility of using the ion-exchange resin AD-2 for the complete release of AAS from biological liquids, in particular from human urine. Second, we studied the conditions of carrying out an enzymic hydrolysis of AAS conjugates in biological samples according to temperature and time of the reaction. To release AAS from urine, the resin XAD-2 (size = 30 to 40 mesh) was used. To determine the completeness of AAS sorption in the resin at different intervals of time, a mixture of ^{3}H-norethandrolone, ^{3}H-methandrostenolone, and ^{3}H-testosterone added to urine samples was used. It was established that 5 min after contact with XAD-2, 65 to 70% of ^{3}H-steroid radioactivity appeared in a bound form. In 10 min 85 to 90% of the hormones were sorbed in the resin, and in 15 min the sorption was nearly complete. Thus, by using the resin XAD-2 only 2 to 3% of AAS in urine is not released. The elution of the steroids off the resin is accomplished with ethyl alcohol.

For AAS (and their metabolites) which are secreted from an organism in a conjugated form, enzymic or acidic hydrolysis appears to be the slowest part of sample preparation for analysis. Enzymic hydrolysis takes 12 to 24 hours and acidic hydrolysis takes 18 to 24 hours. We investigated what effect raising the temperature would have on the velocity of the hydrolysis of 19-nortestosterone conjugates and its metabolites using a mixture of the enzymes of β-glucuronidase arylsulphatase.[32] The enzyme hydrolysis of the samples was carried out at temperatures of 37, 50 and 60° within intervals of 0.5 to 8 hours. The content of 19-nortestosterone was determined by means of RIA. Figure 34 shows that a rise in temperature has a considerable effect on the velocity of the hydrolysis of 19-nortestosterone conjugates. The best results were obtained during enzymic hydrolysis at a temperature of 60°. Within 2 hours the splitting of 19-nortestosterone conjugates was complete.

The investigations carried out led to some improvements in the method of preparing the biosamples containing AAS for analysis on a mass spectrometer. As a result of using these methods, it takes only 2.0 to 2.5 hours to obtain a free AAS fraction and 5 hours to prepare the fraction of conjugated steroids in the same form.

Another trend of investigations was associated with searching for methods that can increase the volatility of AAS. The blocking of polar groups in an

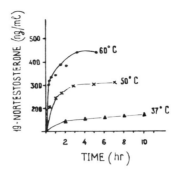

FIGURE 34. The dependence of the efficiency of 19-nortestosterone glucuronide enzyme hydrolysis on temperature.

analyzed steroid molecule by diverse substituents (which forms a part of these groups instead of hydrogen) leads to a reduction in molecular interaction and an increase in substance volatility. Synthesis of the derivatives may also lead to a decrease in nonreversible adsorption due to the change in steroid polarity, the rise in stability, and the increase in the division coefficient. This process must occur with a quantitative result under the condition which excludes decomposition of the substances forming a part of the investigated mixture. The trimethylsilyl (TMS) derivatives, which are formed with a quantitative result and possess a high volatility, are frequently used.[34,35] However, in a number of cases the mass spectra of such derivatives are difficult to interpret. The difficulty occurs when the decomposition is associated with the fragmentation of TMS groups and the molecule's nucleus that often gives smaller intensity peaks of fragmentation ions. In spite of insufficient mass spectra data on most AAS TMS ethers, they possess at least three merits which make their use possible in mass spectrometry analyses. They are formed quantitatively with a high velocity and they possess good GC characteristics. In the mass spectra of 17-O-TMS AAS with different substituents in position 17α: H, CH_3, C_2H_5, the base peaks are m/e = 129, 143 and 157, respectively, which can be used to identify these substances.

For several years the possibility of obtaining various AAS derivatives to use in chromato-mass spectrometry was studied in our laboratory.[39]

For AAS silylation, a mixture of three substances, N-methyl-N-trimethylsilyltrifluoroacetamide (MSTFA), trimethylchlorosilane (TMCS), and trimethylsilylimidazol (TMCI), in the ratio 100:5:2 was used. We succeeded in carrying out the silylation nearly to completion with equal amounts of OH groups and 3-keto group of the steroid for 30 min at 60°C. In this case there was no effect on the 17-oxo group in androsterone or 19-nortestosterone. When obtaining AAS TMS ethers, particular attention was given to the completeness of the reaction with spatially distant OH groups in position 11, fluoxymesterone, and 3-oxo groups. As it turned out, the silylation of the keto groups considerably improved the volatility of steroids. However, the intensity of the ions was slightly reduced to 129, 143, and 157, respectively.

By choosing chromatographic conditions for AAS division, principal attention was paid to the completeness of the division and obtaining the purest chromatographic peak. As a result of the investigations, two kinds of columns were chosen, a WCOT short capillary column with an internal diameter of 0.5 mm and coated with OV-101 (they were used for working in the regime of flow division) and a SCOT microcolumn with an internal diameter of 0.5 mm and coated with SP-2100 (they were used for working in the regime of direct injection). The analyses were carried out on the chromato-mass spectrometer NR-5985 A made by Hewlett-Packard (USA).

There are several possibilities which may be used for AAS determination using GC-MS. First, it is possible to carry out scanning with the sole ion. For instance, the ion with an m/e of 143 is a fragment which usually is obtained by a splitting of ring D of steroid TMS derivatives of 17α-methyl-17β-hydroxy.[40] This method has a rather high sensitivity. It should, however, be taken into consideration that there is a considerable limitation in the specificity which is stipulated by the presence of a large number of AAS having such a fragment. Second, it is possible to carry out a scanning according to a limited number of characterized ions (as a rule 3 to 4) considerably increasing the specificity of substance determination.[36] In combination with GC data on the given steroid retention time, one may extract reliable information about its structure.[40] Lastly, the full mass spectrum, with all registered peaks and their relative intensities, gives a perfect idea of the AAS structure. It is also possible to use a repeated scanning according to the selected ions when a mass spectrum scanning is accompished every several seconds during the sample elution from GC to MS. The results are recorded on a magnetic disc and kept in a computer. Then a mass fragmentogram is plotted according to the characteristic ions and is raised on display and copied.

The mass spectra of some AAS TMS ethers of androstane, androstene and estrene series were investigated. The principal data of the information peaks of AAS TMS ethers are given in Table 28.

Analysis of the results showed a number of moments that limit the wide use of TMS derivatives for AAS analysis. The low intensity of a molecular ion and ions of the type M-15, M-29, M-43, and M-28 for 3,17-TMS androstane, as well as 3,17-di-TMS-androst-4-ens which are similar, was demonstrated. The low intensity of the ions M-90 (M-$(CH_3)_3$SiOH)$^+$, M-90-29 and M-90-15 for the same steroids was also determined. The presence of 17-keto group in 19-norandrosterone and androsterone considerably increases the stability of the molecular ion and the ions M-15, M-30, and M-90-15. The ion peaks 129, 143, and 157 remain the base peaks.

In accordance with these remarks and the data given in Table 28 we offered the order of AAS TMS derivatives chromato-mass spectrometry analysis which

TABLE 28
Retention Time, Formation (%) and Characteristic Ion Intensity of Mass Spectra of TMS-Ethers and Their Metabolites

NN	Series	Name/characterization	RT (min)	%	M+	M-90	R-O-Si(CH$_3$)$_3$
1	Androstane	*Cis*-androsterone-3-β-O-TMS	6.0	100	362.3 (20)	272.2/100)	—
2		19-Nortestosterone-3β-O-TMS	5.0	100	348.2 (24)	258.1 (35)	—
3		Mesterolone-17β-O-TMS	7.3	40	376.2 (20)	286.1 (27)	129 (100)
4		Mesterolone-3ξ,17β-di-O-TMS	7.8	60	448.1 (8)	358.1 (1)	129 (6)
5		Metenolone-17β-O-TMS	8.5	85	374.2 (10)	284.0 (7)	129 (100)
6		Metenolone-3ξ,17β-di-O-TMS	7.8	15	446.3 (40)	356.1 (2)	129 (7)
7		Methylandrostane-3ξ, 17β-di-O-TMS	10.8	100	450.3 (2)	360.2 (4)	143 (100)
8		Oxymetholone-3ξ,17β-di-O-TMS	11.3	100	548.2 (10)	458.1 (1)	143 (26)
9		Stanozolol-17β-O-TMS	12.6	100	400.1 (10)	310.2 (4)	143 (100)
10		Clostebol-17β-O-TMS	13.6	95	394.2 (2)	304.1 (13)	129 (100)
11		Clostebol-3ξ,17β-O-TMS	9.5	5	466.2 (3)	376.1 (5)	129 (100)
12		Methandienone-17β-O-TMS	8.0	96	372.1 (1)	282.1 (23)	143 (100)
13		Methandienone-3ξ,17β-di-O-TMS	8.5	4	444.2 (31)	354.0 (17)	143 (76)
14		Methandienone-6β,17β-di-O-TMS	10.1	100	460.1 (8)	370.2 (3)	143 (100)
15	Androstene	Methylandrostene-3ξ,17β-di-O-TMS	8.5	100	448.2 (6)	358.2 (21)	143 (100)
16		Methyltestosterone-3ξ,17β-di-O-TMS	8.0	100	466.1 (2)	356.1 (6)	143 (55)
17		Testosterone-3ξ,17β-O-TMS	8.2	96	432.4 (8)	342.3 (2)	129 (100)
18		Turinabol-17β-O-TMS	10.7	100	406.2 (1)	316.1 (16)	143 (100)
19		6β-O-TMS-turinabol-17β-O-TMS	11.8	100	494.3 (1)	404.0 (1)	143.1 (100)
20		Fluoxymesterone-3ξ,11β,17β-tri-O-TMS	10.7	80	552.3 (20)	466.2 (15)	143 (100)
21	Estrene	Norethandrolone-3ξ,17β-O-TMS	9.6	95	446.3 (5)	356.2 (10)	157 (100)

are present in human biological liquids. The analysis was carried out in the regime of scanning with full ionic current and masses ranging from 39 to 600 m/e. The analyzed data were recorded on a microcomputer and raised on display initially with the ions 199, 143, 157, then with the ions 136, 141, 274, and so on according to the program created in the laboratory for AAS analysis. Thus, all AAS ions which were present in a nonconjugated form were included. The conjugated AAS were analyzed at first with the ions 272, 333, 348, then with the ions 136, 359, 374 and so on according to the program as well.

When comparing the two methods of GC-MS, scanning with full ionic current and a subsequent data deduction according to characteristic ions and scanning with selected ions demonstrated that the latter method was more sensitive. It was our experience that the application of TMS ethers for AAS analysis by means of mass spectrometry revealed some defects in such volatile derivatives. With a reduction in the concentration of steroids to 1 ng, the peaks in the field of high mass for the lines in which the intensity in the mass spectrum does not exceed 5 to 10% practically disappear. In mass spectra of the substances containing the TMS group, the triplet of molecular ions conditioned by the presence of silicon isotopes ^{29}Si and ^{30}Si at 4.7 and 3.1%, respectively, was observed. Thus, there appeared the necessity for searching for new derivatives of steroids that have higher intensities for heavy ions. By analyzing the methods of obtaining various volatile derivatives of steroids for chromato-mass spectrometry, we could estimate the advantages and the defects of basic reagents used most frequently by AAS derivatization. The application of alkyl- or aryl-methoxylation of 3,17-keto groups led to a modest increase (10 to 30%) of molecular ion outlet. However, it essentially complicates sample preparation for the analysis, and the presence of *cis* and *trans* isomers reduces the sensitivity of the method. The use of nonsymmetric R_1, R_2, and R_3 silyl ethers leads to a rise in the molecular ion intensity, but because of a low potential in the appearance of the ions $(R_1R_2R_3-Si)^+$, the base peak is $(R_1R_2R_3Si-OH)^+$ or $(R_1R_2R_3Si)^+$.

The perfluorated esters of steroids are formed with a high outlet. They possess good GC properties. They are more volatile than the analogous TMS ethers. In mass spectra of perfluorated derivatives the base peaks are $(M-C_nF_{2n+1}-COOH)-R)^+$, where R is a substituent in position 17. The trifluoroacetyl derivatives have good chromatographic properties and also easily react with hydroxylic groups. In our laboratory N-methyltrifluoroacetamide was used for a subsequent study of AAS derivatives. This substance actively reacts and with trifluoroacetylation of steroid hydroxy and keto groups is over within 30 min at 60°. Use of this reagent led to investigating the basic characteristics of mass spectra of 11 AAS trifluoroacetylated (TFA) ethers.

Table 29 shows that TFA derivatives of AAS are more volatile than their TMS analogues. Additionally, by a chromatographic division, the peaks of TFA derivatives are sharper, which increases the sensitivity of the method.

$(M-CF_3COOH-CH_3)^+$ appears to be the base peaks for most TFA derivatives of 17α-methyl-AAS, which considerably increases the sensitivity and reliability of the method since the m/e values of the base peaks and $(M-CF_3COOH)^+$ are suitable for quantification.

The possibility of revealing methandienone in the form of TFA and TMS derivatives in the regimes MID and SIM is shown in Figures 35 and 36.

As the experience of using TFA derivatives for AAS analysis in biological liquids shows, trifluoroacetylation increases the reliability and the sensitivity of chromato-mass spectrometry. It is necessary to note that the absence of a molecular ion, even by the energies of an electron impact of 15 eV and the

TABLE 29
Retention Time, Formation (%) and Characteristic Ion Intensity of Mass Spectra of TFA-Ether and Their Metabolites

NN	Series	Name/characterization	RT (min)	%	M+	M-114/113	M-114-15
1	Androstane	*Cis*-androsterone-3β-O-TFA	4.8	70	386.3 (61)	273.2 (9)	257.2 (13)
2		*Cis*-androsterone-3β-O-TFA	5.6	30	—	272.3 (81)	257.2 (26)
3		19-Norandrosterone-3β-O-TFA	4.2	100	372.1 (100)	258.2 (8)	—
4		Mesterolone-17β-O-TFA	6.6	100	400.0 (36)	287.1 (3)	—
5		Metenolone-17β-O-TFA	7.4	90	398.0 (5)	284.1 (7)	269.1 (17)
6		Metenolone-3ξ,17β-di-O-TFA	5.0	10	494.1 (14)	380.2 (3)	365.1 (17)
7		Methylandrostane-3β,17β-di-O-TFA	4.6	100	—	384.1 (14)	369.2 (100)
8		Oxymetholone-3ξ,17β-di-O-TFA-2-O-TFA-methylene	11.5	100	—	410.0 (13)	395.1 (100)
9		Stanozolol-17β-O-TFA	8.5	7	—	310.4 (13)	295.1 (100)
10		Stanozolol-17β-O-TFA-N-TFA	7.0	93	—	406.2	391.2 (10)
11	Androstene	Methandienone-3ξ,17β-di-O-TFA	9.0	100	—	378 (100)	363.2 (63)
12		Methandienone-3ξ,6β,17β-tri-O-TFA	7.8	10	—	490.1 (24)	475.1 (60)
13		Methandienone-6β,17β-di-O-TFA	4.9	90	—	394.2 (85)	379.2 (100)
14		Methylandrostene-3β,17β-di-O-TFA	3.4	100	—	382.2 (26)	367.2 (100)
15		Turinabol-17β-O-TFA	8.1	80	—	316.1 (18)	301.5 (37)
16		Turinabol-3ξ,17β-di-O-TFA	9.3	20	—	412.0 (20)	397.0 (100)

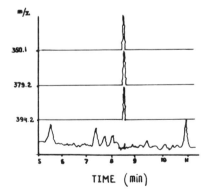

FIGURE 35. Mass-fragmentogram of TFA steroid derivatives of urine containing the basic metabolite of methandienone-6β-OH-methandienone.

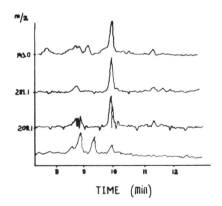

FIGURE 36. Mass-fragmentogram of TMS steroid derivatives of urine containing the basic metabolite of methandienone-6β-OH-methandienone.

absence of common ions for the series 17α-H, 17α-methyl, 17α-ethyl . . . to some extent complicates analysis in the regime of MID.

Thus, based on the material stated in this chapter, one may come to the conclusion that at present there exist technical possibilities for analyzing AAS content and their metabolites in animal and human organisms. As stated above, among the methods which have been practiced on a large scale, the largest preference is given to RIA, HPLC, and GC-MS. In spite of the efficiency and the perspective of using RIA for determining AAS, in the case of needing to determine the structure of their metabolites, an obvious advantage belongs to chromato-mass spectrometry.[16,36,41] By comparing these methods one may find certain advantages and defects in each of them. However, their unification within one laboratory makes it possible to reliably carry out investigations of AAS metabolism at different levels of experimental organization.

REFERENCES

1. **Ambrose, D.,** *Gas Chromatography*, 2nd ed., Butterworth, London, 1971.
2. **Bertsch, W., Jennings, W. O., and Kaiser, R. E.,** *Recent Advances in Capillary Gas Chromatography,* Huethig, Heidelberg, 1981.
3. **Jenning, W. G. and Rapp, A.,** *Sample Preparation for Gas Chromatographic Analysis,* Huethig, Heidelberg, 1983.
4. **Cramers, C. A. and McNair, H. M.,** Gas chromatography, in *Chromatography Fundamentals and Applied Chromatography and Electrophoretic Methods,* Part A, Amsterdam, 1983.
5. **Snyder, L. P. and Kirkland, J. J.,** *Introduction to Modern Liquid Chromatography,* 2nd ed., John Wiley & Sons, New York, 1979.
6. **Hermansson, J.,** Separation of steroid glucuronides by reversed-phase liquid column chromatography, *J. Chromatogr.,* 194, 80, 1980.
7. **Van der Wal, S. and Huber J. F. K.,** Separation of steroid conjugates by high-performance liquid chromatography, *J. Chromatogr.,* 251, 289, 1982.
8. **Krylov, A. I.,** High-performance liquid chromatography of androgen and anabolic steroids: problems and perspectives, in *Muscular Activity and Hormones,* Research Institute of Physical Culture, Leningrad, 1982, 36.
9. **Carvini, A. A. and Di Pietra, M. A.,** High-performance liquid chromatographic analysis of methenolone esters in pharmaceutical formulation, *Int. J. Pharm.,* 13, 333, 1983.
10. **Frischkorn, C. G. C. and Frischkorn, M. E.,** Investigation of anabolic drug in athletics and cattle feed. II. Specific determination of methandienone (dianabol) in urine in nanogram amount, *J. Chromatogr.,* 151, 331, 1978.
11. **Arzamastsev, A. P., Davydov, V. Ya., Gonzales Elizalde, M., Kiselev, A. V., and Rodionova, R. A.,** High-performance liquid chromatography of steroids on silica gel with inoculated phenyl groups, *Chim.-Pharm. J. (USSR),* p. 17, 1983.
12. **Sunde, A. and Lunomo, P. S.,** Separation of 5 reduced androgens by reversed-phase high-performance liquid chromatography, *J. Chromatogr.,* 242, 381, 1982.
13. **Cook, S., Eawlings, N. C., and Kennesy, R. J.,** Quantitation of six androgens by combined high-performance liquid chromatography and radioimmunoassay, *Steroids,* 40, 369, 1982.
14. **Nicolin, B.,** Gas chromatography of steroid hormones, their metabolites and some anabolic steroids, *Arch. Farm.,* 28, 137, 1978.

15. **Smith, D. M. and Steele, J. W.,** Anabolic steroids: chemical rearrangements of oxymetholone, *Can. J. Pharm. Sci.,* 16, 68, 1981.
16. **Cartoni, G. P., Ciardi, M., Giarruso, A., and Rosati, F.,** Capillary gas chromatographic mass spectrometric detection of anabolic steroids, *J. Chromatogr.,* 279, 515, 1983.
17. **Tuinstra, L. G., Traag, W. A., Keukeus, H. J., and Van Mazijk, B. J.,** Procedure for the gas chromatographic-mass spectrometric conformation of some exogenous growth-promoting compounds in the urine of cattle, *J. Chromatogr.,* 270, 533, 1983.
18. **Chmelnitsky, R. A. and Brodsky, E. S.,** *Chromato-Mass-Spectrometry,* Chimiya, Moscow, 1984.
19. **Baba, S., Shinohara, Y., and Kasuya, Y.,** Determination of plasma testosterone by mass fragmentography using testosterone 19-d₃ as an internal standard, *J. Chrom. Biomed. Appl.,* 162, 529, 1979.
20. **Baba, S., Shinohara, Y., and Kasuya, Y.,** Differentiation between androgenous and exogenous testosterone in human plasma and urine after oral administration of deuterium-labelled testosterone by mass fragmentography, *J. Clin. Endocrinol. Metab.,* 50, 889, 1980.
21. **Adleroreutz, H.,** Biomedical application of the mass spectrometry of steroid hormones, *Adv. Mass Spectrum,* 8, 1165, 1980.
22. **Shackleton, C. H. L.,** The analysis of steroids, in *Glass Capillary Gas Liquid Chromatography: Clinical and Pharmacology Analysis,* Jaegr, H., Ed., Dekker, New York, 1981.
23. **Brooks, C. J. W. and Gaskell, S. J.,** Hormones, in *Biochemical Application of Mass Spectrometry,* Wallerm, G. K. and Dermer, O. C., Eds., Wiley, New York, 1980, 611.
24. **Sjovall, J. and Axekson, M.,** Newer approaches to the isolation, identification and quantitation of steroids in biological materials, *Vitam. Horm.,* 39, 31, 1982.
25. **Anderson, A. J. and Warren, F. L.,** Extraction of conjugated androgens from normal human urine, *J. Endocrinol.,* 6, 65, 1951.
26. **Bush, I. E. and Gale, M.,** Extraction and fractionation of steroid conjugates, *Biochem. J.,* 67, 29, 1957.
27. **Hähnel, R. and Chazali bin Abdul Rahman, M.,** Improved gradient elution for the separation of urinary steroid conjugates on DEAE-Sephadex columns, *Clin. Chim. Acta,* 13, 797, 1966.
28. **Sjovall, J. and Axelson, M.,** General and selective isolation procedures for GC/MS analysis of steroids in tissues and body fluids, *J. Steroid Biochem.,* 11, 129, 1979.
29. **Setchell, K. D. R., Taylor, N. S., Adlercreutz, H., Axelson, M., and Sjövall, J.,** The group separation of conjugates of oestrogens using biophilic ion exchange chromatography, in *Research on Steroids,* Klepper, A., Lener, L., Ivan der Molen, H., and Sciarra, F., Eds., Academic Press, London, 8, 131, 1979.
30. **Axelson, M., Sohkberg, B. L., and Sjövall, J.,** Analysis of profiles of conjugated steroids in urine by ion exchange separation and gas chromatography-mass spectrometry, *J. Chromatogr.,* 224, 155, 1981.
31. **Keikkinen, R., Fotsis, T., and Adlercreutz, H.,** Use of ion exchange chromatography in steroid analysis, *J. Steroid Biochem.,* 19, 175, 1983.
32. **Litvinova, V. N.,** An express method of preparation of sample containing anabolic steroids for mass-spectrometry analysis, in *Medical and Doping Control of Athletes,* Leningrad, 1981, 97.
33. **Litvinova, V. N.,** Chemical structure of anabolic steroids and sample preparation for gas chromatography/mass spectrometry analysis, in *Medical and Doping Control of Athletes,* Leningrad, 1981, 103.
34. **Anthony, G. M. and Brooks, C. J. W.,** Characterization of testosterone derivatives and analogues by gas chromatography-mass-spectrometry, *Res. Steroids,* 3, 131, 1968.
35. **Knapp, D. R.,** *Handbook of Analytical Derivatization Reactions,* Wiley-Interscience, New York, 1979.
36. **Donike, M.,** Mass-spectrometric analysis of doping, in *Doping Control of Athletes,* Materials of the International Symposium, October 1979, Moscow, 1980, 61.
37. **Lanito, O., Bjorkhem, J., and Johnston, O.,** Detection and quantitation of stanozolol (Stromba®) in urine by isotope dilution mass fragmentography, *J. Steroid Biochem.,* 14, 721, 1981.

38. **Stan, H. J., Quantz, D., and Abraham, B.,** Gas chromatography-mass spectrometry analysis of anabolic drug residues in meat using electron impact and positive/negative chemical ionization, in *Recent Development in Mass Spectrometry in Biochemistry, Medicine and Environmental Research,* Frigerio, A., Ed., Analytical Chemical Symposia Ser., 7, 338, 1981.
39. **Volkovich, S. V. and Feldkoren, B. I.,** Mass-spectrometric identification of anabolic steroids in biological fluids, in *Medical and Doping Control of Athletes,* Leningrad, 1981, 86.
40. **Laeson, All, Ward, R. J., and Shackleton, C. H. L.,** Mass-spectrometric identification of anabolic drugs, in *Doping Control of Athletes,* Materials of the International Symposium, October 1979, Moscow, 1980, 69.
41. **Durbeck, H. W., Buker, J., Scheulen, B., and Telin, B.,** GC and capillary column GC/MS determination of synthetic anabolic steroids, *J. Chromatogr. Sci.,* 21, 405, 1983.

CONCLUSION

Analysis of the structure and the discovery of AAS active functional groups led to distributing all the AAS which have been synthesized to date into three series: androstane, androstene and estrene. According to the character of the functional groups modified in different positions of the basic steroid skeleton, AAS division was carried out in each of these series. It has been established that by AAS synthesis, of the four types of modifications, testosterone and its derivatives 5α-dihydrotestosterone and 19-nortestosterone are used most frequently. They concern the modifications with C_{17} and C_3, the modifications of ring structure and hydrogen substitution with C_1, C_2, C_4, C_7, C_9, C_{13}, and C_{19} by different radicals. The presence of a steran nucleus in the AAS molecule gives them a number of distinguishable physical-chemical properties, among which are lipophilia and hydrophobia. However, in this case it should be taken into consideration that the formation of differences in hormonal activity is determined by a combination of relatively small modifications in the steroid molecule. By revealing the most significant structural elements that define a selective trend, the strength, and the duration of specific AAS action, one can plan some possible metabolic pathways of these hormones in human organism and experimental animals.

This book examines the processes occurring in target tissues after AAS penetration and successively represents all the events connected with passage of the hormonal signal. In this case principal attention is paid to how these events are linked with the processes of intracellular metabolism. The mechanism of AAS action in an organism includes a successive interaction with transport, receptor and enzyme binding proteins. The characteristics of these proteins interacting with various AAS may essentially differ. A diverse efficiency of the same AAS demonstrated in experiment may depend on absolute values and the ratio of hormone agent towards all three types of specific binding proteins. Skeletal muscle was the tissue type of choice on which the effect of AAS was studied. For comparison we used the tissues of male sex glands. Testosterone and its derivatives actively participate in the regulation of their metabolism. Such an approach had three reasons. First, skeletal muscle constitutes the major mass of an organism and has a number of metabolic peculiarities which differ from other tissues. When moving from a state of rest to carrying out a specific function (muscular contraction), systematic intensification of intracellular metabolism using the existing enzymic system is possible. The high intensity of metabolism in skeletal muscles during physical exercise (which are different according to their character and intensity) remains during the first hours of rest postexercise. One can use such a model for studying the influence of intracellular metabolism on the velocity of passing a hormonal signal into a muscular cell. Various AAS were used as a hormone. Second, the empirical evidence of AAS application in cattle breeding for increasing animal muscular mass demonstrates the existence of some molecular mechanism that ties these events together. Last, until recently skeletal muscle as a target tissue for AAS has not been considered one of the possible sites of action for this group of steroid hormones due to the lack of information on the presence of an indispensable receptor apparatus. Some rare works which appeared in the 1970s were considered to be highly questionable and for a long time they were practically ignored by the preparation of reviews and monographs. Seven years have passed since the publication of Mainwaring's fundamental book that discovered the principal mechanisms of action of androgens in an organism. The skepticism and doubts of this author about the possibility of specific AAS binding in muscular tissue have not been confirmed. On the contrary, the experimental data obtained in our laboratory give convincing evidence as to the presence of a specific binding of various AAS by receptor proteins in cytoplasm and skeletal muscle nuclei. In addition, it was shown that there is an interaction of such a hormone-receptor complex with unique sites of DNA and an intensification of the synthesis of contractile proteins. By using ^{3}H AAS in the method of receptor binding determination, the presence of androgen receptors in cytoplasm and muscular tissue nuclei of different experimental animals was seen. These results were confirmed and expanded in a series of investigations carried out in the laboratories of Gustafsson, Max, Tremblay and others in the years 1980 to 1984.

The androgen receptors in skeletal muscle bind various AAS and therefore may be considered as mediators of hormone action. The affinity of AAS binding to androgen receptors in skeletal muscle and rat prostate was the same. However, the number of binding sites differed essentially. The presence of such receptors in skeletal muscle reflects their hormonal sensitivity and the level of receptors determines a potential direct action of AAS on this tissue. On the basis of these data, the skeletal muscle of a human being or experimental animal may be considered as a target tissue not only for androgens but for AAS as well. Knowledge of the nature of tissue specificity is especially important for realizing the mechanism of AAS action as long as the formation of a wide spectrum of metabolites in target tissues is typical for these steroids.

Study of molecular mechanisms of the hormonal regulation of gene action shows that AAS exert their basic influence on transcription only in the form of hormone-receptor complexes and the association of these complexes with DNA-specific sites in chromatin. At the same time, it is quite possible that the character of the interaction of the hormone-receptor complex is also dependent on higher levels of DNA and DNP structure and on the general organization of chromatin.

By examining the ultimate effects of AAS, it should be taken into consideration that anabolic and androgenic activities which are attributed to these steroids only differ in classification signs and not because these signs or properties concern the steroids. The androgenic effect of AAS in an organism differs from the anabolic effect of the same hormones only according to their localization in tissues and organs and not in their molecular-biological nature. The general molecular mechanism of hormonal regulation of a specific gene activity is the basis of anabolic and androgenic effects of AAS . The specific functions of AAS in an organism are versatile and widely represented in intracellular metabolism of various organs and tissues. AAS positively, but to varying degrees, influence the growth of many tissues. The action of AAS is accomplished through the enzymic apparatus of a target tissue. The concentration of androgenic receptors in tissues and the reactivity of the tissue towards hormone action may change under the influence of AAS. Quantitative changes in the concentration of androgen receptors and the sensitivity of the tissues to AAS, as well as their dependence on sex, age, and functional state, are shown. Active participation of AAS in the regulation of the processes of adaptation of an organism to muscular activity of a different trend was revealed.

The experimental material made it possible to offer the sequence of biochemical processes that ensures the passage of an AAS hormonal signal into the cell in the form of a closed receptor cycle. One can distinguish three peculiarities of the receptor cycle action based on new experimental facts. In recent years more and more data have accumulated showing that the phosphorylation of proteins is a part of a general mechanism of regulation which ties the hormonal and nervous signals with the processes of intracellular metabolism. This concept is based on the possibility that different cellular functions are controlled by protein kinases and protein phosphatases. This has gradually been confirmed by various examples of intracellular regulation including the activation of steroid hormone receptors. It was shown that the process of intracellular receptor activation occurs in the presence of protein kinase and is accompanied by the phosphorylation of a receptor molecule with the participation of ATP. Therefore the process of the interaction of a hormone with a receptor inside the cell is stipulated by the presence of ATP and the state of energy metabolism. The second peculiarity involves the opposite process, that of receptor inactivation, being connected with the dephosphorylation of a receptor molecule in the nucleus under the action of protein kinase. The participation of the processes of receptor protein phosphorylation as an indispensable condition for receptor conversion to an activated state in the presence of a hormone tightly associates the processes of hormonal and intracellular autonomic regulation to a common biochemical mechanism of metabolic control. The third peculiarity shows the possibility of the existence of a closed receptor cycle in the cell nucleus. The presence of free receptors, hormones, protein kinases and protein phosphatases not only in the cytoplasm but also directly in the cell nuclei creates the necessary conditions for the formation of a hormone-receptor complex.

Thus, the possible models of two receptor cycles participating in AAS transport are examined. The first, a large receptor cycle, includes receptor phosphorylation and activation, hormone-receptor complex formation in cytoplasm, and the translocation of such a complex to the cell nucleus. After interaction with chromatin and the activation of specific genes, the hormone-receptor complex is released, the receptor is subjected to dephosphorylation, and hormone dissociation occurs. The receptor and the hormone come back to the cytoplasm and they are able to interact anew with the participation of ATP and protein kinase. The second cycle, a small receptor cycle, proposes carrying out of a phosphorylation process, where receptor activation and hormone-receptor complex formation occur directly in the nucleus with the participation of a nuclear form of the receptor proteins. Interaction of the hormone-receptor complex with chromatin, subsequent dissociation, dephosphorylation and hormone-receptor complex disintegration in the nucleus also occur. The presence of free nuclear receptors and a hormone, as well as the possibility of receptor phosphorylation, make such a model of receptor cycle well-founded.

The experiments carried out by different authors show that the intensity and the character of AAS metabolism depend on the modification of their chemical structure as well as on the enzymic systems of human and experimental animals ensuring the catalysis of the transitions. In the first stage of the biotransformation, AAS participates in the reactions of oxidation, reduction, and hydrolysis. Later on there occurs the formation of more polar hydrophilic metabolites in the reactions of conjugation, with sulphuric and glucuronic acids, which are excreted from the organism in the same form. The basic processes of AAS biotransformation are catalyzed with various enzymic systems which are concentrated in the endoplasmic membranes of liver hepatocytes. Due to the variety of AAS chemical structures, essential differences in the degree of interaction with blood transport proteins and receptor protein target tissues make us examine the common molecular mechanism of AAS action with a certain amount of prudence. The multiplicity of methods of AAS hormonal effects is supposed to be due to a receptor functional heterogeneity. The possibility of the existence of receptors which differ in a number of physical-chemical properties has been confirmed experimentally. The appearance of active metabolites with a higher affinity for androgen receptors in the process of AAS biotransformation may also lead to the ultimate hormonal effect. The phenomenon of the multiplicity of an endocrine regulation may be examined as alternative means of AAS action in muscular tissue. It is manifested in the metabolic control of each tissue with the hormone complex. The effect of several AAS on the level of hormone growth is a good example.

Recently our notions about the basic functions of AAS and metabolism in an organism have become more precise and extensive. However, the participation of AAS in the regulation of intracellular metabolism ensuring the development, the growth, and the reduction of a cell remains one of the major problems which is of interest to many specialists. It is evident that new information on the molecular mechanisms of steroid hormones including AAS will emerge in the near future. It will ensure that the use of these hormones in clinical medicine will be more rational.

INDEX